Ashwagandha

Ancient Secrets Revealed

Ryan T. Scott

Table of Contents

Introduction

Have you ever found yourself wondering if a natural elixir exists that not only promises to revitalize your health but also can reconnect you with the wisdom of ancient wellness traditions? In our constant quest for wellness in a pill, we often overlook the treasures that nature has been holding in plain sight. Among these natural marvels stands *ashwagandha*, an herb with roots deeply entrenched in traditional medicine and an intriguing name that hints at its many potent properties.

The journey that led me to ashwagandha was like many others—a search for something more than I could find in traditional health and medicine. My discovery of ashwagandha was serendipitous, born out of a personal health challenge that conventional medicine could not address without significant side effects. It was during this period of exploration and desperation that ashwagandha presented itself, not just as a supplement, but as a bright light. The turning point came when I witnessed a remarkable transformation in my well-being—not just physically, but mentally and emotionally, evidence of ashwagandha's ability to impart the strength and vitality of a horse.

This book is born out of a desire to share with you the untold story of ashwagandha, to peel back the layers of mystery surrounding this ancient herb and present a clear, concise guide to harnessing its benefits. Through a blend of scientific research, personal narratives, and cultural insights, we will explore the many sides to and uses of ashwagandha, from its role in reducing stress and anxiety to enhancing physical endurance and mental clarity.

Together, we will confront the skepticism that often shadows herbal remedies. The skepticism is not unfounded—after all, the market is rife with products of dubious quality and exaggerated claims. However, this book will arm you with the knowledge to distinguish the genuine from the fake, emphasizing the importance of quality, sustainability, and ethical sourcing in choosing ashwagandha supplements.

As we discover and get to know ashwagandha together, I invite you to keep an open mind and heart. Ashwagandha is more than just a supplement; it is a pathway to understanding the symbiotic relationship between man and nature, a testament to the infinite wisdom and power of traditional medicine. With its tremendous potential and healing abilities, ashwagandha has the power to positively change lives. Now, let's explore how this ancient herb can help lead us to a healthier way of living.

Chapter 1

History is chock full of botanical marvels, each with its tale of discovery, reverence, and utilitarian value that has, over millennia, ingrained itself into various cultures and medicinal practices. Among these, ashwagandha holds a distinctive place—not just for its broad-spectrum therapeutic attributes, but for its venerable history that offers a unique vantage point into the human relationship with natural remedies. Ashwagandha's history is more than simply a chronicle of an herb's utility; it's a strong example of how traditional knowledge, when preserved and propagated, can offer numerous insights and solutions to contemporary wellness challenges.

Unveiling Ashwagandha: A Historical Overview

Ashwagandha's Origins

The genesis of ashwagandha's journey can be traced back to the ancient texts of Ayurveda, written more than 3,000 years ago, when it was celebrated as a potent *rasayana*—a term denoting substances that rejuvenate the body, enhance longevity, and promote mental and physical health. Its botanical name, *Withania somnifera*, encapsulates its dual capabilities: *Withania*, likely derived from the name of the English botanist Henry Witham; and *somnifera*, from the Latin for "sleep-inducing," highlighting its sedative properties. However, in the vernacular, it is known as *ashwagandha*, which in Sanskrit translates to "the smell of the horse," an allusion not only to its distinct aroma but also to the vitality and strength it bestows upon people.

Cultural Significance

Ashwagandha has long been revered in Ayurvedic medicine, not just for its therapeutic prowess but as a symbol of harmony and balance. It was believed to embody the very essence of holistic healing, combining physical well-being with spiritual and emotional health. This reverence was not confined to the Indian subcontinent. Throughout history, ashwagandha has permeated various cultures, each adopting and adapting its use, indicative of the herb's versatile applicability and the universal quest for natural, holistic healing modalities.

Evolution Over Time

From its roots in ancient Ayurvedic texts, ashwagandha's journey through the ages has been marked by a gradual but significant transformation—from a local herb to a globally recognized supplement in the health and wellness market. This transition was not merely a function of globalization but proof of the growing acknowledgment and validation of traditional medicinal practices by contemporary science and medicine. Today, ashwagandha is at the forefront of the adaptogenic revolution, a key player in the movement advocating for natural, noninvasive remedies to combat the stresses of modern life, enhance physical performance, and support overall health and longevity.

Historical Anecdotes

The lore surrounding ashwagandha is as rich and varied as its applications. One notable account involves its use by ancient warriors and athletes to bolster energy and stamina, a practice mirrored in today's sports nutrition and wellness strategies. Another intriguing narrative comes from its role in royal Ayurvedic treatments, where it was incorporated into regimens designed to ensure the longevity and vitality of the rulers, elevating its status in traditional healthcare practices.

As we learn more about ashwagandha's history and cultural significance, take a moment to reflect on the broader implications of this herb's enduring legacy. Consider the following questions, jotting down your thoughts and observations:

- How does the story of ashwagandha's evolution from a local herb to a global wellness phenomenon mirror broader trends in the acceptance and integration of traditional remedies in modern healthcare?

- In what ways can the principles of balance and harmony, central to ashwagandha's role in Ayurvedic medicine, be applied to contemporary wellness practices?

- Reflect on a personal or observed experience in which a return to natural, holistic remedies provided a solution where modern medicine fell short. What insights does this experience offer about the potential role of traditional knowledge in addressing today's health and wellness challenges?

This exercise serves not only as an opportunity to engage more deeply with the colorful history of ashwagandha but also as a prompt to consider the broader implications of integrating traditional wisdom with contemporary health practices. The story of ashwagandha, from its ancient origins to its place in modern wellness, is a compelling narrative that invites us to re-examine our relationship with nature and the potential of natural remedies to enrich our lives.

Ashwagandha in Ayurveda and Traditional Medicine

At the heart of Ayurveda lies the pursuit of balance—a state where the body, mind, and spirit align, creating optimal health and longevity. This ancient holistic healing system, originating from the Indian subcontinent, categorizes the human constitution into three primary life forces or doshas: Vata, Pitta, and Kapha. Each individual is understood as a unique blend of these doshas, with health being the natural byproduct of their equilibrium and disease a manifestation of their imbalance. It is within this context of Ayurvedic medicine that ashwagandha finds its revered place, not merely as an herb but as a foundation of vitality and well-being.

Ashwagandha's role in Ayurvedic practices is fascinating and unique. Classified as a Rasayana, it is hailed for its rejuvenating properties, an herb capable of propagating the vigor and strength of a stallion. The Rasayanas are esteemed for their ability to promote longevity, enhance cognitive function, and fortify the body against the ravages of age and disease. Ashwagandha, with its adaptogenic qualities, stands out among them, with its impressive ability to modulate the body's stress response as well as suffuse it with strength. This adaptogenic prowess is not a mere anecdotal tribute but is backed by a rich history of traditional use and modern scientific validation, underscoring its integral role in Ayurvedic wellness.

When placed alongside other herbs within traditional medicine, ashwagandha distinguishes itself through its broad-spectrum efficacy. Ginseng, for instance, shares the adaptogenic mantle with ashwagandha, yet the latter's ability to induce a state of calm and support restful sleep while simultaneously energizing the body delineates its unique place. Similarly, while turmeric is celebrated for its anti-inflammatory properties, ashwagandha's capacity to enhance muscle growth and recovery showcases its versatility. This comparative analysis does not diminish the value of other herbs but, rather, illuminates ashwagandha's multifaceted nature, offering a holistic approach to wellness that is both preventative and curative.

The integration of traditional ashwagandha applications into contemporary wellness and medical practices is where ancient wisdom and modern science overlap—not as a means to devalue any advances in contemporary medicine but to enrich it with venerable holistic alternatives. When looking at mental health, for instance, where the limitations of pharmacological interventions become evident in their side effects and dependency risks, ashwagandha offers a gentler, yet effective, approach to managing anxiety and depression. Its use in enhancing athletic performance and supporting recovery also reflects this overlap, where ancient tradition and modern medicine can learn to coexist and even work together to create effective solutions.

This combined effect of the old and new is emblematic of a broader shift toward a more integrative approach to health and wellness. It recognizes the limitations inherent within siloed medical practices and the potential of traditional remedies, like ashwagandha, to bridge these gaps. The adoption of ashwagandha in stress management programs, cognitive enhancement protocols, and holistic therapies underscores a growing understanding and acknowledgment of its value—not just as a supplement but as a crucial factor in creating a comprehensive wellness strategy. This trend reflects a paradigm shift, where the dichotomy between traditional and modern medicine gives way to a more collaborative, inclusive approach to health care, one that values the empirical alongside the experiential, the scientific alongside the spiritual.

In this context, ashwagandha has emerged as more than a relic of the past; its relevance has grown, and modern medicine is catching on to the benefits of traditional medicine. From where it emerged, in Ayurveda, to where it lies today, in modern health stores and even pharmacies, ashwagandha has managed to prove its worth and show us that the past and present can come together to create amazing things. Let's keep reading and see what science and research have to teach us about this botanical marvel.

The Science Behind Ashwagandha: What Research Says

Proving itself under great scientific scrutiny, ashwagandha has not only been a subject of casual observation, but many modern research methods have examined and scrutinized it, giving us useful information about its properties and effects on human health. The proliferation of studies dedicated to unraveling the mysteries of this ancient herb speaks to a growing acknowledgment within the scientific community of its potential role in health and wellness. This rise in research seeks to teach us how ashwagandha interacts with human physiology, illuminating its therapeutic benefits and mechanisms of action.

Clinical Studies and Findings

A multitude of studies have methodically charted the effects of ashwagandha on various aspects of human health, from its impact on stress and anxiety to its potential to enhance physical performance and cognitive function. For instance, randomized controlled trials have consistently shown significant reductions in stress and anxiety levels among participants taking ashwagandha supplements, compared to placebo groups. These findings are not isolated but, rather, they reoccur time and time again, suggesting a consistent effect that can benefit anyone and everyone.

Research has illuminated ashwagandha's role in improving muscle strength, body composition, and recovery times, positioning it as a valuable supplement for athletes and physically active individuals. Similarly, emerging studies on cognitive health have revealed promising results regarding ashwagandha's ability to improve memory, attention, and executive function, offering hope for its application in age-related cognitive decline and other neurodegenerative conditions.

Understanding the Evidence

Translating scientific jargon into a more casual vernacular makes it infinitely easier for individuals to connect with and understand the benefits of ashwagandha. For instance, when studies mention ashwagandha's ability to modulate the body's stress response, they refer to its impact on the hypothalamic-pituitary-adrenal axis, a complex network that governs our reaction to stress. By inhibiting the production of cortisol, the body's primary stress hormone, ashwagandha offers a natural means to restore balance and promote a state of calm without the side effects associated with conventional anxiolytics.

This demystification of scientific findings is crucial—not only for creating a deeper understanding of ashwagandha's benefits but also for empowering individuals to make informed decisions about their health and wellness. When people are able to make these informed decisions and understand their options, the true value of all this research becomes incredibly apparent.

Skeptical Viewpoint

Skepticism, far from being a detractor, is a vital component of the scientific process, a tool for refining our understanding and ensuring that conclusions are not drawn from a place of bias or incomplete information. In the context of ashwagandha research, skepticism has brought about a closer examination of study designs, sample sizes, and the quality of ashwagandha extracts used, revealing undeniable variability in results, which further brings about a need for interpretation.

Critics and skeptics point out that while the body of evidence supporting ashwagandha's benefits is growing, gaps remain in our understanding, particularly regarding the long-term effects, optimal dosages, and mechanisms of action. This critical perspective doesn't undermine ashwagandha's potential so much as highlight the importance of continued rigorous research, ensuring that its use is grounded in solid empirical evidence.

Future Research Directions

Looking forward, the future of ashwagandha research is bursting with potential, calling scientists to explore what were previously unexplored components of this herb. Key among these is the investigation of ashwagandha's effects on specific health conditions, such as autoimmune disorders, cancer, and metabolic syndrome, where preliminary studies have suggested potential benefits. Another promising possibility is the exploration of ashwagandha's synergistic effects with other natural compounds, offering the possibility of enhanced efficacy and broader applications.

Moreover, as our understanding of genetics and personalized medicine advances, the opportunity arises to examine how individual variations in genetic makeup affect responses to ashwagandha, paving the way for tailored wellness plans and strategies that can maximize the herb's benefits. This future research, while building on the foundation laid by current studies, holds the promise of not only deepening our understanding of ashwagandha's therapeutic potential but also of incorporating it with various forms of modern healthcare solutions.

Given all this examination and increased understanding of the herb, the scientific community stands on the threshold of a new era in ashwagandha research, working together to enhance understanding and unravel its complexities. By combining the historical knowledge of ashwagandha as a traditional healer with modern scientific inquiry, we can learn more about its benefits for so many different ailments; it also teaches us the value of studying the past so that we can move forward and improve on what we have to offer and potentially help people in greater numbers.

Decoding the Active Compounds: Withanolides Demystified

At the heart of ashwagandha's therapeutic power lies a myriad of phytochemicals, among which withanolides take center stage. These naturally occurring steroids, unique to the nightshade family of plants to which ashwagandha belongs, represent the nexus of the herb's health-promoting effects. The variety of molecules within ashwagandha highlights nature's many creative and healing abilities, a sophisticated ensemble of compounds meticulously engineered by evolution to offer resilience and vitality.

Withanolides, in their structural complexity, serve as molecular architects, constructing and modulating pathways within the human body to allow for healing, balance, and rejuvenation. Their mode of action is both intricate and expansive, interfacing with the body's cellular machinery to mitigate stress, combat inflammation, and protect against cellular damage. Through a series of biochemical interactions, withanolides exert a normalizing influence on physiological processes, gently coaxing the body back to a state of equilibrium. This modulation is particularly evident in their ability to attenuate the stress response, reducing cortisol levels and enhancing mental clarity and focus.

The function of withanolides within ashwagandha is marked by variability, a reflection of the herb's adaptability to different environmental conditions. Not all ashwagandha is created equal; the concentration and composition of withanolides can fluctuate significantly across various strains and growth conditions. This variability underscores the importance of understanding the origin and cultivation practices of the ashwagandha one chooses—these factors directly influence the potency and efficacy of the final product. This variety challenges researchers and consumers alike to discern between different ashwagandha offerings, keeping an eye out for quality and authenticity.

The extraction and formulation of withanolides from ashwagandha roots and leaves are processes that blend tradition with technology. Traditional methods, practiced and perfected over centuries, gently coax these potent compounds from the plant matrix, preserving their integrity and bioactivity. Modern extraction techniques have refined this process, using solvents and methodologies that maximize yield and purity. Yet, formulation involves far more than extraction—it is, in fact, a careful addition of withanolides into supplements and health products designed for optimal absorption and efficacy. This utilization of science and tradition transforms simple ashwagandha into the many magical forms in which it graces our shelves—from capsules and powders to tinctures and teas.

The exploration of ashwagandha's bioactive makeup, particularly its withanolide content, is more than academic science; it's an almost philosophical journey into understanding how this ancient herb interacts with the complex biology of the human body, a chance to learn more about the interactions between natural compounds and our health.

The Botany of Ashwagandha: Understanding Its Growth and Cultivation

Speaking in simple botanical terms, ashwagandha presents itself not merely as a plant but as living proof that nature can and will adapt over time. This small, woody shrub, with its characteristic green leaves and vibrant red berries, thrives under conditions that lesser species would never survive in. Its ability to flourish in the harsh, dry soils of the Indian subcontinent speaks to some sort of evolutionary wisdom, a knack for survival that has implications far beyond mere botanical interest.

The physical characteristics of ashwagandha—its height reaching up to 75 centimeters; its dull, green leaves; and its small, bell-shaped flowers—offer only a superficial glimpse into its biological complexity. The real magic lies beneath the surface, where we can't see it, but we know that there's a complicated network of roots there. It is within these unseen roots that ashwagandha stores its potent withanolides, the very compounds that help to create those sought-after therapeutic properties. The lifecycle of ashwagandha, from germination to maturity, unfolds over the course of a year, a brief span in which it must complete its cycle of growth, reproduction, and seed dissemination.

Cultivation practices for ashwagandha fall somewhere between tradition and innovation. For centuries, farmers in India have planted seeds with the onset of the monsoon and harvested the roots as the dry season approaches, understanding that keeping with natural cycles improves results and ensures the optimal development of the plant, which, in turn, maximizes the concentration of bioactive compounds in its roots. Modern agricultural techniques have built upon these traditional practices, turning to science to increase yield and quality. Soil amendment, irrigation strategies, and organic pest-control measures are judiciously applied, balancing the need for productivity with the goal of preserving the natural integrity of the plant.

The influence of geography on the properties of ashwagandha cannot be overstated. The plant's native habitat, the arid regions of India, offers a unique set of environmental conditions—dry soil, minimal rainfall, and high temperatures—that ashwagandha has adapted to over thousands of years. When cultivated in regions with differing soil compositions, rainfall patterns, and temperatures, variations in the plant's phytochemical profile are observed. These geographical nuances are critical for cultivators and consumers alike, as they directly impact the plant's therapeutic efficacy. Understanding this, cultivators must choose their sites with care, favoring locations that mimic ashwagandha's natural habitat to ensure the highest quality harvest.

Sustainable farming practices are imperative when attempting to cultivate ashwagandha. This change over time reflects a growing awareness of the environmental and social responsibilities that accompany agricultural production. Sustainable agriculture, in the context of ashwagandha cultivation, encompasses a range of practices designed to minimize environmental impact while ensuring the health and safety of farmers and communities. Crop rotation, organic farming methods, and water conservation techniques are necessary to preserve soil health, reduce dependency on chemical inputs, and safeguard water resources. Moreover, sustainable cultivation practices ensure the long-term availability of ashwagandha, protecting this valuable resource for future generations.

Ashwagandha's botany, from its physical attributes and lifecycle to its cultivation and the influence of geography, makes crystal clear the importance of integrating human science with the natural world. This combination helps to preserve the fragile ecosystem as well as encompass a holistic view of agriculture that respects and preserves this fragile balance of man and nature. In this light, ashwagandha stands not only as a source of health and wellness but as a symbol of the symbiotic relationship between humanity and the natural world, a reminder of the delicate interdependencies that sustain life on our planet.

Quality Matters: Identifying High-Grade Ashwagandha

If you want to find the finest ashwagandha, you need to pay attention and be a little picky. This process requires that you understand the markers that denote high-quality ashwagandha, markers that are both visible to the naked eye and hidden within the chemistry of the plant. The concentration of withanolides, the primary bioactive compound, serves as the foremost indicator of quality. High withanolide content translates to enhanced potency, offering more pronounced therapeutic benefits. Yet, our search for quality does not end with chemical composition alone. The physical attributes of ashwagandha, including the color and texture of the root, offer many clues. A high-quality root presents a light, creamy hue and a firm, yet fibrous, texture, characteristics that reflect optimal growing conditions and careful harvesting practices.

Navigating the market for ashwagandha supplements requires more than a cursory glance at physical and chemical markers; you also want to double-check its certifications and testing. Products that have undergone rigorous testing and have been awarded certifications for purity and potency stand out in a crowded marketplace. These certifications, from recognized bodies like the United States Pharmacopeia (USP) or the Non-GMO Project, inform the consumer that this product has been vetted and meets stringent quality standards. The process of certification encompasses a detailed examination of the product, from the sourcing of raw materials to the manufacturing processes, ensuring that what reaches the consumer is both safe and effective.

However, ashwagandha products certainly have their pitfalls. Misleading marketing tactics often cloud the truth, presenting challenges for those in search of genuine quality. You will find many claims of superior potency or exclusive properties, but they frequently fall short under scrutiny. The savvy consumer must learn to navigate these claims with a critical eye, digging a bit beneath the surface to see the real substance. You want to read labels with precision, discern fact from fiction, and distinguish marketing fluff from genuine quality indicators. The ingredient list, concentration of withanolides, and presence of fillers or additives become focal points in this evaluation, guiding the consumer in making informed choices.

But there's more. Beyond the markers of quality and the marketing morass lies the pivotal issue of sourcing. Ethically sourced ashwagandha cannot guarantee quality, but you want to go that route to support environmental and social responsibility, and you are more likely to find a high-quality product this way. Ethical sourcing ensures that the ashwagandha is grown in conditions that respect the natural cycle of the plant, adhere to sustainable farming practices, and provide fair compensation to the farmers and communities involved in its cultivation. This approach to sourcing has a direct impact on the quality of the ashwagandha, as plants grown under ethical and sustainable conditions are likely to yield higher concentrations of bioactive compounds, including withanolides. Furthermore, ethical sourcing contributes to the sustainability of the ashwagandha supply, ensuring that this valuable herb remains available for future generations.

A careful, discerning consumer will find their way through the confluence of quality, certification, marketing, and sourcing. They will have a deep appreciation for the nuances that define high-quality ashwagandha and a commitment to making choices that are informed, ethical, and sustainable. Sticking with an ethically sourced product leads the consumer to so much more than its therapeutic benefits; it leads to a deeper connection with the very essence of ashwagandha, rooted in tradition, science, and a deep respect for nature.

Ashwagandha's Global Journey: From Local Herb to Global Superfood

Ashwagandha has managed to make a name for itself within global health consciousness with remarkable finesse, which is impressive given the constantly changing and evolving wellness trends on the market. It's worth noting that this little herb we call ashwagandha was once exclusive to the dry climate of India; it then found its way into Ayurveda, and now, after traveling across the world through science, you can find it at the health store as well as see books like this one on the market. Not bad.

The spark that ignited ashwagandha's rise in popularity beyond its native soil can be traced back to a growing disillusionment with conventional medicine's approach to chronic conditions and a collective desire for natural, holistic healing modalities. As researchers began to validate the anecdotal benefits of ashwagandha with empirical evidence, its appeal broadened, finding its place among both alternative and conventional medicines. This validation was not merely a nod to its efficacy but a recognition of its potential to complement modern therapeutic practices, offering a gentler, more integrative approach to wellness.

The cultural exchange that gave rise to ashwagandha's global journey is akin to a dialogue between traditional knowledge holders and scientific communities. This dialogue, enhanced by respect and curiosity, has propelled ashwagandha from relative obscurity to global recognition. You could say this serves as a reminder that the pursuit of health and well-being is a universal language and that, through this exchange, ashwagandha has become more than an herb. You could say that it has served as a bridge between Ayurveda and ancient practices and modern science and that both have become better for it.

However, the burgeoning global demand for ashwagandha has cast a spotlight on the communities where this herb is traditionally grown. The surge in interest has brought economic opportunities to these regions, offering farmers and cultivators a lucrative market for their harvests. This influx of demand has the potential to transform local economies, providing a sustainable source of income and encouraging the preservation of traditional cultivation practices. But this opportunity is not without its challenges. The pressure to meet global demand can strain natural resources, necessitating a careful balance between cultivation and conservation. It is within this context that the role of sustainable farming practices is critical, ensuring that the cultivation of ashwagandha contributes to the well-being of local communities while preserving the ecological balance.

The potential economy of traditional herbs like ashwagandha, while opening avenues for cultural exchange and economic growth, also presents ethical considerations that warrant some understanding. As ashwagandha transitions from a local herb to a global superfood, questions arise about the ownership of traditional knowledge, the risk of biopiracy, and the fair compensation of indigenous communities. These considerations need to exist because making ashwagandha a commodity requires a strong sense of responsibility and equity. The communities at the heart of this little herb need to be recognized and rewarded for the role they play in creating it.

In grappling with these challenges, the global community faces a critical choice: to go down the path of exploitation and environmental ruination or choose the path that embraces ethical sourcing and sustainability. The latter honors ashwagandha's heritage. This choice will determine not only the future availability of ashwagandha but also the integrity of the global wellness movement. The adoption of fair trade practices, the investment in sustainable agriculture, and the recognition of traditional knowledge as a collective heritage are steps toward a future where ashwagandha continues to thrive, both as an herb and as a symbol of a more integrative, respectful approach to health and healing.

As ashwagandha continues to gain global popularity, it invites us to reconsider our relationship with nature, to explore the synergies between different healing traditions, and to work toward a future where wellness is accessible, sustainable, and shared across cultures. This multifaceted journey offers a glimpse into the potential of traditional herbs to enrich our lives—not only physically but culturally and environmentally, as well.

Safety First: Understanding Dosages and Side Effects

With its myriad benefits, ashwagandha requires understanding dosage and possible side effects. Next, we will look at recommended dosages and possible side effects and interactions.

Recommended Dosages

Determining the right amount of ashwagandha depends on your desired outcomes and how your body physiologically responds to it. Understanding that dosages are easily adaptable, daily amounts typically span 300–500 milligrams of high-concentration extracts, an amount formulated for general wellness objectives—stress reduction, better cognition, and so on. For more specific health goals, such as improving endurance or mitigating insomnia, this dosage might be adjusted upward, with clinical guidance to help gauge tolerance and achieve the best dosage.

Potential Side Effects

While ashwagandha is lauded for its safety profile, it, like any herb or medicine, has a list of potential side effects, albeit rare and generally mild. These may manifest as gastrointestinal discomfort, drowsiness, or in some instances, an allergic reaction characterized by itching or rash. Such occurrences, while rare, serve as a reminder of the importance of starting with lower dosages and observing one's reactions. Moreover, someone with a thyroid condition needs to proceed with caution, as the herb can have a potent effect on the endocrine system. It requires simple monitoring and possible dosage adjustments.

Interactions With Medications

The intersection of ashwagandha with pharmaceutical interventions warrants careful examination, given the herb's potential to interact with certain medications. Notably, its calming properties could amplify the effects of sedatives, while its influence on blood sugar levels necessitates some caution for those treating diabetes. Similarly, due to its capacity to affect blood pressure, individuals on antihypertensive drugs should approach ashwagandha with caution. The fact that many interactions with ashwagandha are possible means simply that you need to consult with a professional before starting your regimen.

Special Populations

Pregnant and breastfeeding women should proceed with caution and definitely consult with a medical professional. At present, there simply isn't enough data to know for certain how safe it is and at what dosage ashwagandha is best used. The same holds true for individuals with autoimmune diseases such as rheumatoid arthritis or lupus, conditions marked by an overactive immune system; they might find ashwagandha's immunomodulatory effects to be a double-edged sword, necessitating medical oversight.

The bottom line is that exploring dosages, side effects, and interactions requires mindfulness and informed decision-making. Integrating herbal supplements such as ashwagandha needs to be considered with great care and caution as well as a commitment to understanding and respecting the intricacies of this ancient herb, ensuring that its benefits are harnessed in a manner that prioritizes safety and well-being.

Ashwagandha Through the Ages: Use Across Lifespan

Throughout our lives, from the tender, young years to the wiser, older ones, we are faced with nonstop health challenges of one kind or another as well as a myriad of opportunities for growth. As it happens, ashwagandha can offer us a wide variety of benefits, presenting itself as an herbal ally, able to offer support at various stages along the way.

Adolescence is marked by rapid growth and hormonal upheaval, a constant whirlwind of emotions, and, of course, puberty. Ashwagandha can serve as a stabilizer, helping to mitigate the stressors that accompany this phase of life. Its capacity to modulate stress hormones offers a grounding effect, potentially easing the transition through puberty and creating a sense of equilibrium amidst the whirlwind of change. Ashwagandha can continue to help young ones as they step into adulthood, building a career and a family life, enhancing focus and endurance and offering an oft-needed natural boost of energy.

Later, in our golden years, ashwagandha can help us maintain or even improve our health, vitality, and cognitive function. Ashwagandha's potential to bolster memory and cognitive agility offers the elderly hope, a natural adjunct to aging gracefully. Moreover, its anti-inflammatory properties may play a role in alleviating the discomforts of aging joints, while its influence on energy levels helps counteract the lethargy that often accompanies advancing years.

Navigating the dosage and form of ashwagandha across our various life stages requires a tailored approach, attuned to the changing needs of the body. For younger individuals, lower dosages and forms that integrate easily into daily routines, such as powders blended into smoothies, might be preferable. Adults, balancing the demands of work and family, may lean toward more concentrated forms, such as capsules or tinctures, offering convenience without compromising efficacy. In the later years, a gentle reintroduction through teas or mild supplements can provide the support needed without overburdening a system that might be managing multiple health considerations.

There is much discourse on ashwagandha's role in life and longevity, keeping in mind the blending of ancient wisdom and modern research. Theories have speculated that the herb's adaptogenic capabilities can help reduce the impact of stress on the body, a factor intimately linked with aging. Exploratory studies hint at ashwagandha's potential to enhance telomerase activity, an enzyme associated with cellular aging, suggesting a fascinating avenue for future research on its role in promoting a longer, healthier life. Whereas in ancient times, ashwagandha was esteemed as a rejuvenator, a harbinger of vitality and longevity, its use permeating all stages of life with the promise of enhanced well-being, today, this traditional reverence converges with a growing body of scientific evidence, affirming its timeless appeal and expanding its numerous benefits to address the multifaceted health challenges of the modern world. It is this bridging of knowledge that explains ashwagandha's continued and enduring relevance—its ability to adapt to the needs of every generation serves to prove its value to us all.

The Environmental Impact of Ashwagandha Cultivation

As ashwagandha's role in holistic wellness has grown over the years, the ecological footprint of its cultivation casts a long, intricate pattern across the landscapes it inhabits. Nurturing ashwagandha from seed to harvest is not without its environmental considerations, encompassing a broad spectrum from water consumption to the transformation of land. The symbiosis between this revered herb and the ecosystems that support its growth invites a closer examination, revealing the delicate balance between agricultural productivity and ecological stewardship.

Precise management of water resources is a necessary component of cultivating ashwagandha, regardless of its adaptability to arid climates. In regions where water scarcity poses a perennial challenge, irrigation becomes a matter of strategic importance. The plant's resilience to drought conditions offers a semblance of reprieve, yet the optimization of water usage through drip irrigation and rainwater-harvesting techniques underscores a commitment to minimizing waste. This approach not only ensures the sustainable growth of ashwagandha but also safeguards local water reserves, preserving them for future generations.

Where ashwagandha cultivation is concerned, the expansion of its farming has led to the transformation of landscapes, with fields once dedicated to food crops now swathes of green dedicated to this medicinal herb. This shift, while economically viable for farmers, raises questions about food security and biodiversity. Farming ashwagandha, if unchecked, risks diminishing soil health and reducing the genetic diversity of local plant life. Herein lies the impetus for integrating crop rotation and polyculture practices, strategies that maintain soil vitality and encourage a peaceful, healthy coexistence of multiple species.

The growing demand for ashwagandha has not gone unnoticed by conservationists, who voice concerns over the strain on wild populations. The allure of wild-harvested ashwagandha, considered by some to be more potent, has led to overharvesting in certain areas, threatening its natural regeneration. This situation highlights the need for sustainable harvesting practices that allow for the replenishment of wild ashwagandha, ensuring that its collection does not outpace its growth. The cultivation of ashwagandha under controlled, sustainable conditions offers a practical alternative, reducing pressure on wild populations while meeting global demand.

Amid these environmental considerations, the role of sustainable initiatives holds great promise and hope. Across the globe, farmers, researchers, and corporations are joining forces to implement practices that align with the principles of sustainable agriculture. These initiatives range from the adoption of organic farming methods, which eschew synthetic pesticides and fertilizers, to the implementation of integrated pest management systems that rely on natural predators to control pests. Such practices not only reduce the ecological footprint of ashwagandha cultivation but also enhance the quality of the final product, creating a win-win scenario for both the environment and consumers.

The bottom line is that consumers are the biggest players in ashwagandha's ecological future. By opting for ashwagandha sourced from farms that prioritize sustainability, consumers can drive demand in a direction that supports ecological balance and social equity; we can wield considerable influence over farming practices, which in turn affects market trends. It may seem like a small contribution, but in the grand scheme of things, making good choices can cause a ripple effect across the supply chain, eventually greatly influencing producers. As we navigate the complexities of ashwagandha cultivation, let us tread lightly upon the Earth, mindful of the legacy we leave for the future generations who will walk these paths long after us.

Chapter 2:

Ashwagandha—A Lifeline in the Age of Anxiety

In a world that never sleeps, stress and anxiety have become as ubiquitous as the air we breathe. Amid our constant restlessness, ashwagandha has become curative, helping us combat the stress and anxiety we have become so accustomed to. Between research-driven science and centuries of natural use, ashwagandha has arrived and remains a remedy rather than a modern quick fix.

Stress, Anxiety, and Ashwagandha: A Natural Solution

Efficacy in Reducing Stress

Ashwagandha's ability to reduce stress is backed by a myriad of clinical studies. A notable investigation published in the *Journal of the American Nutraceutical Association* details how subjects consuming ashwagandha experienced a significant reduction in stress levels, quantified by a marked decrease in cortisol, the body's stress hormone. This reduction was not merely statistical but visible in tangible improvements in the subjects' quality of life, thereby proving ashwagandha's potential role in helping people manage their stress levels.

Mechanism of Action

Ashwagandha's adaptogenic properties offer a fascinating glimpse into its mechanism of action. Adaptogens, a unique class of herbal compounds, offer resilience against the multifaceted challenges of stress by modulating the body's stress response systems. In short, ashwagandha tunes up the hormones and neurochemicals involved in the stress response, ensuring that the body's reaction to stressors is balanced and appropriate. This modulation is pivotal, as it prevents the overexertion of the adrenal glands and creates a state of equilibrium, shielding the body from the potentially damaging effects of chronic stress.

Personal Stories

Consider the scenario of Anna, a high school teacher. Anna has felt weighed down by the demands of work and the constant pressure to meet expectations. After incorporating ashwagandha into her daily routine, she notes a discernible shift in her ability to manage classroom challenges and administrative tasks—her anxiety levels have been noticeably reduced. On a day-to-day basis, Anna feels much better, like she can take on her pressures with a better attitude and more energy. This anecdote mirrors countless others, reflecting a wide variety of experiences in which ashwagandha has provided solace and strength, allowing people to live better lives and navigate their pressure with grace.

Guidance on Usage

If you are considering ashwagandha to help you with your stress levels, practical guidance on its usage is indispensable. An effective starting point is a daily dosage of 300–500 mg of a high-concentration ashwagandha extract, ideally taken with meals to enhance its absorption. However, you need to view this as a foundational guideline rather than a rigid prescription, as the optimal dosage may vary based on individual factors and specific health goals. A period of observation and adjustment is recommended, allowing one to calibrate the dosage to their unique physiological response. Moreover, consistency is key, as the benefits of ashwagandha accrue over time, necessitating regular intake over several weeks to fully manifest its stress-alleviating effects.

As we have mentioned, the confluence of scientific evidence, mechanistic insights, and personal testimonies paints a compelling picture of ashwagandha's efficacy in the battle against stress and anxiety. Continued research and countless personal experiences serve to support its potential as a natural, holistic solution to the many challenges of modern life.

Sleep Solutions: How Ashwagandha Promotes Restful Nights

Many people find themselves unable to quell their thoughts and give in to sleep at night, during life's quiet hours. Ashwagandha again comes to the rescue, ready and willing to help you overcome your insomnia and quiet your mind.

The Role of Ashwagandha in Enhancing Sleep Quality

Dedicated investigations into ashwagandha's influence on sleep patterns reveal promising trends in our great quest for sleep. These studies, meticulously designed to quantify the herb's impact, consistently report improvements in both sleep onset latency—the time it takes to fall asleep—and the overall quality of sleep among participants. Sleep is just as much about quality as it is about quantity. Such findings provide a solid foundation for ashwagandha's esteemed status as a soothing, restorative agent, capable of nurturing the body's natural rhythms and guiding it toward a state of restful equilibrium.

Biochemical Underpinnings of Ashwagandha's Sedative Effects

While ashwagandha's sedative properties are observable in research outcomes, they are rooted in complex biochemistry. Triethylene glycol, a component isolated within the herb, plays a pivotal role, gently engaging with the nervous system. This interaction does not blanket the brain in a fog of forced stupor but gently soothes neurotransmitter activity toward relaxation and sleep readiness. It's a subtle recalibration of the body's internal mechanisms, one that respects the natural cadence of waking and sleeping, aligning physiological processes with the external cues of nightfall.

Weaving Ashwagandha into Nighttime Rituals

Incorporating ashwagandha into your evening routines transforms it from a mere supplement into a ritualistic aid that cues the body for sleep. Small, thoughtful adjustments to these routines can amplify ashwagandha's effectiveness. A cup of warm milk infused with ashwagandha powder, consumed a short while before bed, works as both a physical and symbolic gesture toward winding down. The warmth of the milk, mixed with the grounding properties of ashwagandha, creates a concoction that soothes the body and quiets the mind. This ritual, when repeated, becomes a signal to the self, a preparation for the shift from activity to rest, enhancing ashwagandha's natural propensity to gently calm you down.

Narratives of Transformation: Ashwagandha and Improved Sleep Patterns

The narratives of those who have found solace in ashwagandha are as varied as they are inspiring. Consider the account of a writer, plagued by insomnia that often accompanies his intended bouts of creativity, for whom night after night he is restless and unable to sleep. With ashwagandha, he is gradually able to sleep not just longer, but also better, which serves to improve every aspect of his waking life.

Another tale comes from a nurse, her sleep patterns fragmented by the irregular hours of her profession, who discovered in ashwagandha a steadying influence, giving her the ability to get the sleep she needs, even with her relentless and irregular schedules.

These stories, each unique in its context, share a common theme: ashwagandha's ability to share its holistic—physical, mental, and emotional—properties and help you find not just a sleep aid but a better ability to balance your life.

Boosting Immunity With Ashwagandha

The modern era, with its rapid pace and heightened exposure to environmental stressors, demands more from our biological defenses, placing unprecedented stress on the immune system. Within this context, ashwagandha's role as an immunomodulator is not merely beneficial but becomes indispensable in its ability to promote resolve and health. Its ability to subtly enhance the various structures of the body is nothing short of amazing.

Strengthening the Immune System

Scientific research into ashwagandha's capacity to bolster immunity reveals a fascinating interaction of compounds and biological mechanisms. Research delineates ashwagandha's efficacy in upregulating the activity of macrophages, guardians of the immune system, known for their prowess in engulfing pathogens. This enhancement of macrophage activity signifies a more vigilant immune surveillance, ensuring a swift and thorough response to microbial invasions. Furthermore, ashwagandha has been shown to increase the production of immunoglobulins, proteins that play a critical role in identifying and neutralizing foreign invaders such as viruses and bacteria. This dual action, both at the cellular and molecular level, exemplifies ashwagandha's comprehensive approach to immune support, fortifying the body's defenses from within.

Antioxidant Properties

Beyond its direct immunomodulatory effects, ashwagandha's rich array of antioxidants contributes significantly to its immune-boosting capabilities. These antioxidants, by scavenging free radicals, mitigate cellular damage and reduce oxidative stress, a condition known to compromise immune function. The reduction in oxidative stress not only preserves the integrity of immune cells but also enhances their efficiency, ensuring that the immune system operates at its peak. This aspect of ashwagandha shines a light on the body's interconnected systems and its positive effects on them.

Combination With Other Immune Boosters

Ashwagandha's potential to synergize with other natural immune enhancers opens avenues for creating holistic wellness regimens. For instance, the combination of ashwagandha with vitamin C–rich foods or supplements can enhance the body's antioxidant defenses, offering a defense against oxidative stress and pathogenic threats. Similarly, integrating ashwagandha with probiotics, the beneficial bacteria that colonize the gut, may enhance gut-associated lymphoid tissue's function, a crucial component of the immune system. This potent combination of ashwagandha with other immune-supportive elements showcases its ability to support those other elements and offer a multidimensional approach to wellness.

Real-Life Applications

The real-world implications of ashwagandha's immune-boosting effects are as diverse as they are impressive. Consider the experiences of individuals living in regions prone to seasonal flu outbreaks, for whom regular ashwagandha supplementation has helped them immensely in maintaining health during peak flu seasons. By enhancing their immune resilience, ashwagandha has enabled them to get through these long, cold seasons with fewer incidences of illness—or, in cases where infections occurred, to experience milder symptoms and quicker recoveries. Similarly, for those stressed out by contemporary life, from the relentless pace of professional commitments to the environmental stressors of urban living, ashwagandha has served as a protective shield, fortifying their immune system against the potential dampening effects of chronic stress.

In each instance, ashwagandha proves that it's more than a supplement; it's an effective herb that supports overall well-being. Its impact is not isolated to the immune system but extends to enhancing vitality, reducing stress, and promoting balance across bodily systems. This holistic influence is particularly relevant in times of heightened stress— whether physical, emotional, or environmental—when the immune system's efficacy is critical. Through regular ashwagandha usage, individuals arm themselves with a natural, time-tested adjunct to health, one that supports not just the immune system but the entire spectrum of well-being.

Keep in mind that ashwagandha is not a panacea. It's a meaningful supplement that supports the body's defenses and nurtures health and stamina from within. Its subtle effects aid the body's strength and function. As we've said, in today's modern landscape, ashwagandha represents the effective combination of nature and medicine. With each person who incorporates it into their lifestyle, we can see strengthened immunity, enhanced well-being, and a greater connection to the natural world.

Ashwagandha for Physical Performance and Recovery

Ashwagandha has become a handy and powerful tool in athletics, where the limits of human potential are continuously tested and redefined. This ancient herb has transitioned into sports science, revealing its impressive capacity to enhance both physical performance and recovery.

Enhancing Athletic Performance

Investigations into ashwagandha's impact on athletic performance have illuminated its role in augmenting strength and stamina—two elements all athletes need a lot of These studies depict a significant increase in muscle mass and strength in individuals supplementing with ashwagandha, a finding that clearly relates to athletics—in particular, weight training and competitive sports. Ashwagandha's ability to naturally elevate testosterone levels, enhancing muscle growth and recovery, as well as its adaptogenic properties, which contribute to improved stamina, give it a great advantage in any athlete's desire to attain peak performance.

Reducing Muscle Damage

The rigors of intense physical activity invariably subject the body to muscle damage and inflammation, a tool that can impede recovery and performance. Here, ashwagandha's anti-inflammatory and antioxidative properties play a crucial role in mitigating cellular damage and accelerating the repair processes. By attenuating the markers of muscle damage, such as creatine kinase, ashwagandha aids in faster recovery, ensuring athletes can return to their training regimens with minimal delay. This attribute, deeply rooted in the herb's bioactive compounds, underscores its value not merely as a supplement for enhancing performance but as a vital component of the athlete's recovery protocol.

Usage in Sports Nutrition

The incorporation of ashwagandha into sports nutrition has seen a pronounced trajectory, propelled by growing awareness of its benefits among athletes and fitness professionals. This trend has seen ashwagandha make its way into pre-workout blends and recovery formulations, chosen for its natural efficacy and alignment with the holistic wellness ethos that increasingly characterizes sports nutrition. The preference for ashwagandha in these formulations is not arbitrary; an expanding body of research has validated its role in improving physical performance and supporting recovery, offering a natural alternative to synthetic supplements.

Testimonials From Athletes

Ashwagandha's impact on athletic performance and recovery is vividly brought to life through the testimonials of sports professionals and fitness enthusiasts. These personal accounts offer a window into the real-world implications of ashwagandha supplementation, going beyond science and humanizing it with their success stories. From marathon runners who have experienced enhanced endurance and reduced post-race recovery times to bodybuilders who report significant gains in muscle strength and mass, the stories are as varied as they are compelling. Each testimonial can convince just about anyone of ashwagandha's adaptogenic and restorative powers, reinforcing its standing as an indispensable asset in the athlete's toolkit.

The fact that athletes and fitness professionals, as well as people studying and practicing sports medicine, have embraced ashwagandha as a natural, holistic way to enhance their performance and studies speaks to its empirical evidence and many positive personal experiences. For those looking for a natural alternative to enhancing their capabilities, ashwagandha stands miles above the rest, proving that combining modern-day science with herbs and traditions of the past can create a successful approach to endless enhancements to our lives.

Balancing Hormones Naturally With Ashwagandha

Within the intricate world of human physiology, hormones emerge as the silent, yet strong, director of bodily functions—from the subtle shift in moods to the complex processes of growth and metabolism. It is here, within this incredible factory working toward hormonal balance, that ashwagandha can take over gently, carefully guiding the whole system toward equilibrium. As with our many previous examples, it offers a natural approach and addresses the root causes of whatever may be ailing you.

Regulating Thyroid Function

The thyroid gland, a modest entity in the human body, holds sway over a vast domain, dictating the functionality of metabolic processes with its secretions. Ashwagandha, in its capacity as a natural endocrine modulator, has been demonstrated to wield influence over thyroid hormone levels, nudging them toward a state of balance. This influence is particularly poignant for those grappling with hypothyroidism, where ashwagandha's intervention spurs an increase in the production of thyroid hormones, catalyzing a reawakening of metabolic functions that were languishing and not doing their jobs. Through their years of methodical research, the scientific community has begun to look deeper into ashwagandha's impact on thyroid health; signs point to its ability to help restore the glands that are causing so much trouble.

Effects on Adrenal Health

Parallel to the thyroid, the adrenal glands engage in their own hormone production, pivotal in the body's response to stress. Ashwagandha steps onto the scene with a dual role; it tempers the overproduction of cortisol, the stress hormone that, in excess, creates imbalance, and revitalizes adrenal function, which can falter under the weight of chronic stress. This rejuvenating effect on the adrenals embodies ashwagandha's adaptogenic essence, offering respite to the weary glands and fortifying the body's resilience against the pressures that besiege it. The recalibration of adrenal output that follows ashwagandha supplementation is inspiring and hopeful for those who need help with chronic stress and hormonal imbalances.

Fertility and Reproductive Health

Where reproductive health is concerned, ashwagandha again can help restore hormonal imbalances, which in this case is good news for fertility. For women, ashwagandha's intervention promises an alleviation of the symptoms that accompany conditions such as polycystic ovary syndrome (PCOS), ushering in a restoration of ovulatory cycles and hormonal profiles. Men, in parallel, witness an augmentation of seminal quality and a bolstering of testosterone levels, both factors integral to reproductive vitality. These potential effects underscore ashwagandha's role not merely as a supplemental aid but as a promising support to reproductive health and fertility.

Evidence and Personal Experiences

Ashwagandha's talent for balancing hormones and enhancing fertility is enriched and backed by myriad personal accounts as well as years of scientific study and evidence. Accounts of couples who, in their infertility battles, turned to ashwagandha and found hope in its potential, illuminate the path for others facing similar challenges. These stories, each unique yet unified by ashwagandha's curative benefits, create a compelling argument for its inclusion in reproductive health regimens. Coupled with rigorous scientific investigations that endlessly study ashwagandha's hormone-modulating effects, these personal accounts offer a multidimensional perspective on the herb's capabilities, bridging the divide between traditional wisdom and contemporary medical understanding.

Once again, ashwagandha stands as an icon of the healing power of nature, offering a key to unlock the door to hormonal balance and well-being. Its role in regulating thyroid and adrenal function and in nurturing fertility and reproductive health is not just a matter of historical record or scientific observation but a living legacy that continues to unfold. As research looks deeper into the mechanisms of ashwagandha's action and more individuals share their stories of healing, this ancient herb's story continues to grow richer and more powerful, offering hope for those living with the challenges of hormonal imbalance.

Cognitive Benefits: Enhancing Memory and Brain Function

Deep in our minds, where memories weave through our thoughts and cognition gets us through the day, ashwagandha comes to the rescue, guarding and maintaining mental acuity. This ancient herb again comes to the rescue, revealing a plethora of cognitive benefits. After all, as we age, modern life takes its toll on our minds as we manage an onslaught of information and a need to concentrate amidst the disquiet of nonstop distractions. Ashwagandha stands out as a shining star for those who are struggling with memory fog, lack of clarity, and difficulty maintaining focus.

Improving Cognitive Function

The evidence supporting ashwagandha's role in bolstering memory, sharpening focus, and accelerating cognitive speed is both rich and compelling. Diverse studies punctuate the scientific literature, identifying the herb's efficacy in enhancing various facets of cognitive function. One such investigation describes its ability to improve immediate and general memory in individuals, casting a light on its potential to strengthen mental clarity. Another study elucidates ashwagandha's capacity to elevate cognitive speed, a boon to the brain's processing capabilities, enabling quicker assimilation and retrieval of information. This variety of cognitive enhancements speaks to ashwagandha's multidimensional impact, positioning it as an invaluable ally in our desire and need for greater mental acuity, especially as we age.

Neuroprotective Properties

Beyond the immediate augmentation of cognitive function, ashwagandha's influence extends to neuroprotection, offering a shield against the oxidative stress that preys upon the brain. The herb's arsenal, rich in antioxidants, mounts a defense against the free radicals that catalyze cellular degradation, a frontline resistance that may curtail the advance of neurodegenerative diseases. This protective mantle is not only a barrier but an active participant in the preservation of neural integrity, creating an environment where neurons thrive, unburdened by the shadow of oxidative damage. Such neuroprotective prowess suggests a potential for ashwagandha to stand as a defense against the decline of cognitive function, guarding the gateways of memory and thought against the encroachments of age and disease.

Application in Daily Life

The integration of ashwagandha into daily life heralds a new chapter for individuals seeking to nurture their cognitive health across a spectrum of settings, from the academic to the professional and the personal. In academic contexts, students find in ashwagandha a natural adjunct to enhance learning, memory retention, and exam performance, a study aid that supports the mind in grasping complex concepts and recalling vast tracts of information. Professionals, meanwhile, harness ashwagandha's capacity to boost focus and cognitive speed, an edge in the fast-paced world of business and innovation, where mental agility is necessary. Beyond these domains, ashwagandha serves as a companion in the personal journey toward lifelong learning and mental wellness, supporting hobbies, interests, and the simple joy of a vibrant, active mind.

Success Stories

Ashwagandha's cognitive benefits are rife with success stories, narratives that breathe life into the data and research findings. Consider the tale of a novelist, for whom writer's block became her enemy, the empty page taunting her and making her life miserable. With ashwagandha, the fog lifted, revealing a clear path where words flowed with newfound ease, her cognitive faculties reinvigorated. Another account tells of an aging professor who, facing the twilight of his career, grappled with the dimming of his once-sharp memory. Ashwagandha became his solace, a means to reclaim the keen edge of his intellect, allowing him to impart wisdom with the clarity that had defined his teaching for so many years. These stories serve as validation of ashwagandha's impressive impact and its influence on the mind's capacity to remember, focus, and think, once again, with clarity.

Where cognitive enhancement is concerned, the pursuit of mental clarity and longevity speaks to the core of human aspiration. In this context, ashwagandha emerges as a key player. Its role in improving memory and brain function serves beyond its traditional known uses, finding resonance in the heart of modern science and the lives of those it touches. With each study that unveils its benefits and each story that celebrates its impact, ashwagandha reaffirms its place as a cornerstone of cognitive health, a natural ally in the quest for a vibrant, focused, and resilient mind.

Ashwagandha and Heart Health: A Holistic Approach

The human heart beats at the core of our health and wellness, a symbol of life's rhythm and vitality. Amidst the cacophony of modern existence, with its relentless pace and myriad stressors, the heart often bears the brunt, any hints of its distress drowned out until they become undeniable calls for attention. Herein lies the silent promise of ashwagandha, offering its strength to fortify the heart—not through obvious and loud proclamations but through the quiet assurance of its healing embrace.

Cardiovascular Benefits

Ashwagandha's contribution to heart health is a multifaceted look at science and exploration and the benefits this trusty herb can provide. Among the myriad benefits, its role in modulating cholesterol levels stands prominent, confirming its capacity to navigate the lipid landscape, lowering the markers of bad cholesterol while gently elevating the good. This lipid modulation, critical in the prevention of atherosclerosis, positions ashwagandha as a guardian of arterial health, its actions a subtle nudge toward cardiovascular health and vitality. Moreover, the enhancement of circulation, another feather in its cap, ensures a free flow of life's essence throughout the body, each heartbeat enriched by the nourishment it delivers and the wastes it banishes. This dual action, targeting both the quality of blood and its unimpeded flow, portrays a picture of holistic heart health, improved and encouraged by ashwagandha.

Stress and Heart Health

The link between stress reduction and heart health, illuminated by the calming influence of ashwagandha, reveals the depth of its impact. When suffering from or dealing with stress, the heart flutters and falters, its rhythm disrupted by the surge of adrenaline and cortisol, heralds of the fight-or-flight response. Ashwagandha, in its role as an adaptogen, can calm this storm, tempering the adrenal response—and with it, easing the burden on the heart. The correlation between lowered stress markers and reduced blood pressure, a direct benefit of ashwagandha's intervention, tells the story of lowering the risk of heart disease as well as reinforces the interconnectedness of emotional well-being and physical health. Every step toward this connection is a step toward a healthier heart.

Integrating With Heart-Healthy Lifestyles

As with any herbal contribution to good health, ashwagandha is at its most beneficial with the other elements of a heart-healthy lifestyle. In the confluence of diet, rich in fruits, vegetables, and whole grains; exercise; and stress management, ashwagandha finds its best, most effective rhythm. This integration, a blend of nature's wisdom with human endeavor, crafts a lifestyle where the heart thrives, encircled by the protective embrace of holistic wellness. Ashwagandha does not overshadow but complements, its presence a subtle enhancement to the lifestyle choices that form the bedrock of cardiovascular health. The suggestion to sprinkle a bit in your morning smoothie or a capsule at dinner becomes not just advice but a call to action, a step toward embracing a life where the heart beats strong and free.

Ashwagandha's many positive testimonials mix data with experience, allowing for a realistic impression of users' experience with this vibrant herb. Narratives unfold, each unique yet unified in its essence, of lives touched and transformed by the subtle power of this herb. Take, for example, a middle-aged man, his life a juggling act between professional demands and personal commitments, his heart health neglected and placed at the bottom of a long list of priorities. With ashwagandha, the scales tipped back to balance, his cholesterol levels a reflection of this newfound equilibrium, a victory not just for him but for the family that cherishes his presence. Another story speaks of a woman in her later years, her heart weathered by time yet resilient, finding in ashwagandha a companion in her journey toward maintaining cardiovascular health, her vitality restored. These stories, each a small part of ashwagandha's impact, resonate with a truth that transcends numbers and data, a truth lived and felt, one heartbeat at a time.

In physiology, where the heart reigns supreme, ashwagandha offers its strength, not as a panacea but as a partner in the pursuit of wellness, a holistic ally in the journey toward a life lived with vitality and joy. Its benefits, a blend of ancient wisdom and modern science, beckon to those who seek not just to survive but to thrive, each heartbeat a symbol of health, each breath a testament to the amazing power of nature's healing touch.

Weight Management and Metabolic Benefits of Ashwagandha

In the complicated world of metabolic health, where the balance of energy intake and expenditure dictates the ebb and flow of weight, ashwagandha once again guides the body toward where it needs to go—in this case, a state of equilibrium. This ancient and potent herb unfolds its leaves to reveal a wide array of benefits that extend into weight management, a domain where modern dilemmas intersect with timeless solutions. Ashwagandha, in its essence, offers a bridge across this divide, its roots anchoring the promise of metabolic harmony in the fertile ground of scientific validation and human experience.

Influence on Metabolism

The metabolic rate, a hard-working element of digestion where calories are consigned to bodily functions, finds in ashwagandha a catalyst, a means to increase and improve energy consumption. This modulation of metabolic rate is not a mere acceleration but an optimization, wherein ashwagandha's adaptogenic properties calibrate energy expenditure to the needs of the body, enhancing fat oxidation without tipping the scales toward depletion. Such an effect, illuminated by metabolic studies, suggests a pathway through which ashwagandha supports weight-loss efforts—not through drastic measures but through a gentle recalibration of metabolic processes, creating an environment where weight management becomes a natural outcome of bodily balance.

Appetite and Cravings

Appetite is often weight management's most formidable foe. Here, ashwagandha's role goes beyond the physical, striving to simplify and improve the psychological interplay between stress and eating behaviors. By mitigating the various levels of stress that often precipitate emotional eating, ashwagandha curtails the origins of the cravings, aligning appetite with the genuine needs of the body rather than the fleeting whims of stress-induced appetites. This readjustment of appetite, underscored by research into ashwagandha's impact on stress hormones, offers a respite to those stuck in the cycles of binge eating and dietary remorse, all of which is a step toward cultivating healthier eating habits grounded in mindfulness and physiological need.

Synergy With Diet and Exercise

In the confluence of dietary choices and physical activity, where nutrition and exercise merge, ashwagandha finds its stride, enhancing the efficacy of each while paving a synergistic path to metabolic health. The integration of ashwagandha with a balanced diet, rich in the nutrients that fuel metabolism, amplifies the body's capacity to derive energy efficiently from food, optimizing nutrient uptake and utilization. Concurrently, ashwagandha bolstering of physical stamina enriches the exercise experience, not merely by extending the threshold of fatigue but by enhancing the body's recovery post-exertion, ensuring that each session of physical activity contributes to the goal of weight management at its maximum level. This orchestration of diet and exercise, mediated by ashwagandha, embodies a holistic approach to metabolic health, a strategy where the sum of efforts exceeds their individual contributions.

Personal Weight-Loss Journeys

The narrative of ashwagandha's effect on weight management is vividly chronicled in the stories of individuals who have lived and dealt with the constant challenges of weight loss with this herb as their companion. These accounts, diverse in their backgrounds yet unified in their challenges, speak to the transformative potential of ashwagandha. One such story recounts the journey of a woman who, entangled in the web of yo-yo dieting, found in ashwagandha a stabilizing force, a means to anchor her efforts in the calm of reduced stress and balanced metabolism. Her success, measured not just in pounds shed but in the newfound vitality and equilibrium, marks a testament to ashwagandha's role in weight management. Another narrative recounts the tale of a man for whom physical activity had become a chore, an undertaking that offered little joy. With ashwagandha, the vigor returned to his steps, and exercise changed from a burden to a source of strength, his weight loss journey reignited with a sense of accomplishment and renewal.

In these stories, as with countless others, ashwagandha's contribution to weight management emerges not as a solo traveler but as one of many herbal and medicinal choices, each piece integral to the whole. The herb's influence on metabolism, appetite, and the synergistic augmentation of diet and exercise are rife with possibility, all part of a scenario where weight management aligns with the broader objectives of health and well-being. Ashwagandha helps anyone struggling with weight loss to embrace a more nuanced understanding of balance and harmony of body and mind in the pursuit of better health.

The Anti-Inflammatory Effects of Ashwagandha

As part of the body's response to injury and infection, inflammation sometimes protects and sometimes creates further ailments. With the help of contemporary science and research, ashwagandha clearly possesses a potent anti-inflammatory power. This revelation is not a mere footnote in herbal medicine but an evolving chapter that underscores the herb's relevance in mitigating inflammation, a common point in a spectrum of chronic conditions.

Combating Inflammation

The scientific community, armed with its traditional blend of curiosity and rigor, has illuminated the pathways through which ashwagandha exerts its anti-inflammatory effects. The herb's arsenal, rich in withanolides, targets the molecular morasses involved in inflammation, offering a countermeasure to the body's sometimes overzealous immune response. These withanolides inhibit the activity of nuclear factor kappa B (NF-κB), a protein complex pivotal in the transcription of inflammatory genes. By curbing the excess production of pro-inflammatory cytokines, ashwagandha acts not with the blunt force of pharmaceuticals but with the precision of a scalpel, fine-tuning the immune response to foster healing rather than exacerbate distress.

Applications for Chronic Conditions

The implications of ashwagandha's anti-inflammatory action extend far beyond the acute phases of swelling and pain; it also can greatly and positively affect chronic inflammatory conditions. Arthritis, with its hallmark of joint inflammation and degradation, emerges as a prime candidate for ashwagandha's intervention. The herb's capacity to alleviate joint pain and swelling, hallmarks of arthritis, has been documented, offering sufferers a glimmer of reprieve. Beyond the joints, ashwagandha's reach spans to inflammatory bowel disease (IBD), where it soothes the gut's inflamed lining, and to the nebulous inflammation associated with metabolic syndrome, offering a multipronged approach to wellness that addresses not just the symptoms but the underlying inflammatory processes.

Daily Dosage and Administration

Understanding ashwagandha's optimal dosages and forms serves to improve its anti-inflammatory benefits. For those seeking to mitigate inflammation, a daily intake ranging from 250 to 500 mg of high-concentration ashwagandha extract is recommended. This dosage, derived from the confluence of traditional use and modern research, serves as a guideline, a starting point from which individual adjustments can be made based on response and specific health objectives. The herb's versatility in any form—be it capsules for convenience or powders for incorporation into smoothies or teas for a soothing ritual—ensures its accessibility to all, allowing for a tailored approach to administration that respects personal preferences and lifestyles.

User Experiences

Individual experiences and stories that animate the herb's benefits beyond the confines of clinical trials further confirm ashwagandha's tremendous and curative impact. Accounts from those who have turned to ashwagandha speak of a softening of chronic pain, a loosening of stiffness in the joints, and a general uplift in well-being.

One story tells of a gardener, her hands gnarled from years of toil and the creeping onset of arthritis, who found in ashwagandha a way to soothe her pain and a companion as she was able to keep working with the dirt she so loved. Another story recounts the journey of an athlete, sidelined by the persistent inflammation of tendinitis, who, with ashwagandha, was able to combat the inflammation and once again enjoy movement in all its forms.

These stories, each a tale of personal triumphs over inflammation's grip, echo the broader promise of ashwagandha. They remind us that within this ancient herb lies not just the potential for physical healing but an invitation to rekindle the body's innate resilience, a collective desire to live fully and embrace life with diminished pain and discomfort.

Managing Chronic Conditions With Ashwagandha

After so many years of traditional use and scientific study, ashwagandha occupies a place of honor, revered not only for its versatility but for its efficacy in managing a wide variety of chronic conditions. This ancient herb has exceeded the expectations of its traditional confines, working with modern science to inspire those suffering from chronic ailments. From diabetes to autoimmune diseases, ashwagandha extends its healing embrace, offering a natural adjunct to the complicated world of modern therapeutics.

The array of chronic conditions that ashwagandha has been able to offer improvement includes so many ailments, from the metabolic dysregulation of diabetes, through the inflammatory pathways of autoimmune disorders, to neurodegenerative conditions like Alzheimer's and Parkinson's disease. This broad-spectrum utility underscores the herb's adaptogenic nature, a unique attribute that enables it to modulate physiological processes, restoring balance and functionality to systems thrown into disarray by chronic disease. The adaptogen's capacity to attenuate stress, a common exacerbator of chronic conditions, further amplifies its therapeutic potential, offering a dual mechanism through which it cultivates wellness and vitality.

The foundation of ashwagandha's therapeutic acclaim rests on a growing compendium of research that illustrates its role in managing and potentially ameliorating chronic conditions. Studies delineate its hypoglycemic effects, highlighting its ability to modulate blood sugar levels in diabetic patients, offering a glimpse into its potential as a natural adjunct to diabetes management. Similarly, research into autoimmune diseases reveals ashwagandha's immunomodulatory capabilities, showcasing its ability to recalibrate the immune system's response, reducing the severity of symptoms and potentially altering the disease's trajectory. This compilation of scientific inquiry, while continually evolving, provides a compelling argument for ashwagandha's inclusion in the management of chronic conditions.

The integration of ashwagandha into an integrative health strategy represents a paradigm shift in the management of chronic conditions, a move towards a holistic approach that can surpass the limitations of conventional treatments. This herb complements pharmacological interventions, offering a natural means to mitigate side effects, enhance therapeutic outcomes, and improve overall quality of life. Its role extends beyond mere symptom management, touching on the root causes of ailments, from metabolic imbalances to immune dysregulation, creating a state of health that is built on the foundation of systemic balance and flexibility. This integrative approach, where ashwagandha operates alongside conventional therapeutics, embodies the essence of holistic healing, a strategy that views the individual as a cohesive whole, where mind, body, and spirit are inextricably linked.

As this chapter in the exploration of ashwagandha's therapeutic versatility draws to a close, you will find that the stories and irrefutable evidence leave a lasting imprint. The herb's broad-spectrum benefits, underpinned by scientific evidence and enriched by personal testimonials, tell a narrative that transcends the confines of traditional and modern medicine, offering a holistic approach to managing chronic conditions. In ashwagandha, we find not just a remedy, but a companion on the path to wellness, a natural ally that complements conventional treatments and creates a state of balance and vitality. This exploration, while highlighting chronic conditions, is but a small piece of ashwagandha's healing potential, a prelude to the continuing journey into the depths of this ancient herb's therapeutic bounty.

Chapter 3:

Establishing Your Ashwagandha Practice—A Step-By-Step Guide

In the quiet predawn hours, when the world is slowly waking up, the day full of potential, the ritual begins. A kettle whistles, steam rises, and the earthy scent of ashwagandha fills the air. This moment becomes more than a routine; it becomes a practice, a daily commitment to wellness and balance. Ashwagandha, revered for centuries for its healing properties, now finds its place in modern health practices—not through grand gestures but through the simple, steadfast repetition of daily use.

In this chapter, we'll focus on the practical, guiding you through the establishment of your ashwagandha practice. This guidance, wrought from traditional and modern wellness strategies, aims to incorporate ashwagandha into your daily routine, ensuring steady, positive benefits for your many years ahead.

Establishing a Routine

As is true with cultivating any practice or skill, consistency gets to the heart of the matter. Consider the morning, the start to every new day, as the ideal backdrop for your ashwagandha intake. The calm of the morning, before things get hectic and complicated, offers a moment of pause, an opportunity to nurture your body and mind with ashwagandha's grounding presence. For those who find the evening more conducive, as the day is winding down, ashwagandha can gently usher in a restful night, its adaptogenic properties balancing the body's stress responses as you drift off to sleep.

Consistency Is Key

The adage "Rome wasn't built in a day" finds resonance in the context of building an ashwagandha practice. The herb's benefits unfold over time, requiring a commitment to regularity. Marking your calendar as a visual reminder or setting a daily alarm can serve as simple yet effective strategies to create a consistent routine. Just as watering a plant requires regular, daily care, each day you continue with ashwagandha is a step toward deeper wellness.

Listening to Your Body

The wisdom of the body holds invaluable insights into the optimization and effectiveness of your ashwagandha practice. Start with the recommended dosage, observing how your body and mind respond over those first few weeks. Some may find a slight adjustment in dosage or timing necessary, a reflection not of a misstep but of the unique dialogue between your physiology and ashwagandha. This process is like tuning an instrument; in this case, the instrument is your body and it seeks harmony and balance that will resonate with your needs and wellness goals.

Integrating Mindfulness

Mindfulness, the art of presence, amplifies the benefits of ashwagandha, creating a synergy that enhances stress reduction and promotes a sense of well-being. Incorporating a brief mindfulness practice—perhaps a moment of focused breathing or a short meditation—immediately before or after taking ashwagandha, anchors its use in a state of heightened awareness. This integration not only enhances the immediate sense of calm and balance but also deepens the overall impact of your ashwagandha practice, each mindful breath sharing its myriad benefits with you.

Interactive Element: Journaling Prompt

Reflect on your initial experiences with ashwagandha. Note any changes in stress levels, sleep quality, or general well-being. Use these observations to fine-tune your practice, adjusting dosages or timing as needed.

Wellness trends ebb and flow with the tide of public interest. Ashwagandha is proof positive of natural healing's enduring power and efficacy. Its journey, from the ancient soils of India to the shelves of modern health stores, mirrors the broader search for balance and wellness in a world marked by constant change. Establishing your ashwagandha practice, steeped in the principles outlined in this chapter, offers not just the promise of individual health benefits but a connection to a tradition that has grown over centuries, a practice rooted in the wisdom of the past yet fully engaged with the needs of the present. As you incorporate ashwagandha into your daily routine, remember that each step, each choice, brings you closer to wellness and lights the way toward a healthier connection with this ancient healing herb.

Ashwagandha Recipes for Beginners: Simple and Affordable

Ashwagandha, with its great many health benefits, naturally invites you to incorporate it into your daily routine. Teas and snacks are no exception. By adding this natural wonder to your diet, in whatever capacity you choose, you are integrating ashwagandha into your daily life, which will help regulate you amid all the hustle and bustle. The following recipes are meant to be simple, despite the immense impact they can have on you and your health.

Smoothies and Teas: Elixirs of Vitality

The morning, with its promise of new beginnings, presents an opportune moment for infusing the day with ashwagandha and its grounding energy. To make a smoothie, a perfect vessel for this herb's many benefits, consider blending a teaspoon of ashwagandha powder with a mix of bananas, spinach, and almond milk—a concoction that blends the herb's earthiness with the natural sweetness of fruit and the creaminess of the milk, creating a beverage that energizes and balances in equal measure.

Similarly, the ritual of tea preparation—steeping leaves, watching the steam rise, and inhaling the aromatic blend—becomes a meditative practice when ashwagandha joins the infusion. A simple ashwagandha tea, requiring nothing more than a teaspoon of the herb's powder combined with hot water, honey, and a slice of lemon, can transform a mundane routine into a moment of tranquility, a pause that can reinvigorate and prepare you for the day's challenges.

Energy Bars: Sustenance on the Go

Given the relentless craziness of contemporary life, finding moments for balanced meals can often elude even the most organized individuals. Ashwagandha-infused energy bars offer a solution, a compact source of nourishment that fits neatly into the chaos of daily schedules. Mixing ashwagandha powder with oats, nuts, seeds, and a binding agent such as honey or maple syrup, then baking the concoction until it solidifies, produces a batch of energy bars that can help you maintain vitality and focus throughout the day. These bars can easily be customized to cater to individual taste preferences, showing, once again, how versatile this herb is and how easy it is to integrate into a fast-paced lifestyle.

Golden Milk: A Prelude to Restful Slumber

As the day winds down, the body and mind begin their descent toward rest. It is in this twilight hour that golden milk, infused with ashwagandha, emerges as a delicious source of relaxation. Combining a teaspoon of ashwagandha powder with warm milk, turmeric, a dash of black pepper (to enhance turmeric absorption), and a sweetener to taste creates a beverage that soothes while it heals. It supports sleep, reduces inflammation, and prepares the body for the regenerative work of night. Its preparation, a ritual that signals the end of day, helps you transition from wakefulness to sleep, slumbering peacefully with the holistic benefits of ashwagandha.

Budget-Friendly Tips: Accessible Wellness

Embracing the healing potential of ashwagandha doesn't need to cost you an arm and a leg; wellness, after all, should elevate, not burden. Sourcing ashwagandha, whether in powder or root form, from local health stores or online platforms that offer bulk purchases can significantly reduce costs. Additionally, incorporating the herb into existing recipes or meals, rather than creating dishes around it, ensures its benefits are realized without requiring elaborate culinary undertakings. The versatility of ashwagandha, compatible with both sweet and savory dishes, from smoothies to soups, allows you to integrate it easily into your routine, showing yet again how versatile and adaptable it is.

These offerings are simple in execution but full of potential to enhance well-being. By mindfully incorporating ashwagandha into your daily routine—in whatever form you prefer—you're connecting to the natural world, reaping benefits from its impact and its ability to soothe, temper, and heal.

DIY Ashwagandha Tinctures and Extracts

The alchemy of transforming ashwagandha from its raw form into a potent tincture or extract encapsulates the essence of proactive wellness. This process brings you closer to its healing properties as you gain a deeper connection to them. Crafting ashwagandha tinctures and extracts at home is a way for you to be self-sufficient in your health care and practices, merging its ancient properties with your modern kitchen.

Step-By-Step Extraction

You can start to create an ashwagandha tincture by gathering roots, the part of the herb rich in withanolides, those precious phytochemicals full of adaptogenic virtues. After cleaning and drying the roots, chop them finely or grind them, awakening the potent compounds nestled within their fibers. Submerge the prepared roots in a solvent, typically high-proof alcohol; you have now initiated the extraction. Over weeks, in a sealed container hidden from light, a transformation unfolds; the alcohol leeches the withanolides from the roots, combining with ashwagandha's essence. Once you have strained it, you have yourself a tincture, a liquid extract that can improve your health

By contrast, extracts are more potent than tinctures; they are created by a more intricate process, where water and alcohol in varying stages coax a concentration of its active compounds from the ashwagandha. This dual extraction method creates a powerful liquid, an embodiment of ashwagandha's healing potential in concentrated form.

Equipment and Ingredients

The tools required for this endeavor are deceptively simple, yet each plays a crucial role. Glass jars with tight-fitting lids safely hold the mixture as it steeps, while cheesecloth or fine-mesh strainers stand ready to separate the solid roots from the liquid essence. Amber bottles, their color a shield against the degradation of light, await the final product, ready to preserve the potency of the tincture or extract. The ingredients, though few, demand careful selection; ashwagandha roots, either fresh or dried, sourced with an eye for quality; and a solvent—alcohol for tinctures, alcohol and water for extracts—chosen for purity.

Storage and Usage Instructions

Proper storage is crucial for preserving a tincture or extract's vitality; amber bottles, with their contents labeled with date and concentration, should remain in cool, dark places, protecting their potency from the damage of light exposure over time.

To fully enjoy and reap ashwagandha's benefits, start by adding one of these preparations a few drops at a time, either in water or tea. Your response to its slowly developing potency will dictate any dosage adjustments you may wish to make going forward. Pay close attention to your responses as you go.

Safety Considerations

When working with tinctures and extracts, safety and cleanliness are crucial. Each step, from the preparation of the roots to the bottling of the final product, must be performed with careful hygiene practices, ensuring that the end result is not only potent but pure. The choice of alcohol, particularly for tinctures, navigates the balance between efficacy and safety, its proof adequate for extraction yet mindful of consumption. By staying attentive to details, you'll have a product that exemplifies ashwagandha's essence, created by you!

Integrating Ashwagandha With Other Adaptogens

Ashwagandha, with its broad spectrum of positive effects, can work on its own, but as part of a collective of herbs, it shines. In this collective, each herb contributes unique strengths—in a concept called adaptogenic synergy, the combined effect of the variety of herbs surpasses the sum of their individual benefits, opening up treatments rich with possibilities for enhanced wellness. Ashwagandha contributes to stress reduction as well as to bolstering immunity, as you know, and it sits at the heart of this integrative approach, ready to be intertwined into this holistic approach alongside its herbal peers.

The alchemy of blending ashwagandha with other adaptogens requires both intuition and insight, understanding the nuanced effects of each herb and listening to the subtle cues of your body. For those seeking to invigorate energy levels, the combination of ashwagandha and rhodiola serves as a potent duo. Rhodiola, with its capacity to elevate stamina and mental clarity, complements ashwagandha's stress-modulating effects, creating a blend that not only energizes but also ensures that this heightened vitality rests on a foundation of balanced stress responses.

Conversely, for individuals cursing their chronic stress and anxiety, ashwagandha finds a harmonious partner in holy basil. Known in Ayurvedic tradition as *Tulsi*, holy basil shares ashwagandha's adaptogenic ability to mitigate stress, yet introduces a unique facet of uplifting mood and spiritual wellness. Together, they form a blend that not only shields the body from the myriad negative effects of stress but also nurtures the mind and spirit, creating a sense of tranquility and resilience.

The art of customizing blends invites a deeper engagement with the world of adaptogens, encouraging a journey of discovery that is as personal as it is therapeutic. This process begins with a reflection on your health goals and challenges, a mapping of the terrain that these botanical allies are enlisted to navigate. From there, the exploration of individual adaptogens—be it the stamina-enhancing cordyceps, the antioxidant-rich goji berry, or the mood-stabilizing schisandra— becomes an exercise in crafting a personalized wellness solution. The preparation of these blends, whether as teas, tinctures, or capsules, becomes a means of healing, each ingredient chosen for its efficacy.

Yet, as with any form of potent medicine, the integration of ashwagandha with other adaptogens requires mindfulness, particularly regarding potential interactions and the importance of moderation. The principle of starting with low doses helps you move carefully, ensuring that the body has the space to adapt and respond without being overwhelmed. This cautious approach, coupled with an attentive observation of the body's reactions, safeguards against the rare but real possibility of adverse interactions, allowing for a gradual increase in dosage as confidence in the blend's effects grows.

Learning about and wading through the vast expanse of adaptogenic herbs, ashwagandha playing its part in healing the body and soul, introduces you to a path to wellness, founded both on ancient tradition and relevant science. The synergy achieved through thoughtful combinations not only amplifies the individual strengths of each herb but also speaks to a deeper truth about health—that it is most fully realized in balance, in the harmonious interplay between various elements of care. In this light, ashwagandha's integration with other adaptogens encompasses body, mind, and spirit, proof of the interconnectedness of life and a reflection on the holistic nature of health. It is a proven strategy for enhanced well-being.

As you navigate and master this terrain, the blending of ashwagandha goes far beyond the act of mixing ingredients; it becomes a form of alchemy, a meaningful process that not only enhances health but also deepens the connection to the natural world. This integration can flourish as a vibrant expression of holistic healing, inspiration for anyone looking to enhance their well-being alongside the rhythms of nature and the wisdom of the ages.

Ashwagandha for Beauty: Topical Uses and Benefits

Where the ancient wisdom of herbalism intersects with the pursuit of aesthetic vitality, ashwagandha is king. Its roots extend their reach into the modern wellness world, offering a natural elixir against the ravages of time and the environment. This section discusses the many varied applications of ashwagandha when incorporated into personal care, spotlighting its potential to rejuvenate, protect, and enhance the skin and hair's natural luster.

Skin-Care Benefits: A Natural Shield Against Time

Dermatology and ashwagandha are powerful allies, wielding their anti-inflammatory and antioxidant properties with precision. The relentless advance of time, coupled with environmental stressors, orchestrates a silent war against the skin, rapidly advancing all signs of aging. In response, ashwagandha mounts a defense, its bioactive compounds mitigating oxidative stress and inflammation, the sneaky instigators of cellular degradation. With this intervention, collagen synthesis flourishes, safeguarding skin's elasticity and delaying the onset of wrinkles. Moreover, ashwagandha's ability to modulate the stress-response system offers protection against the ignoble effects of stress-induced acne, presenting a holistic avenue to dermatological vitality.

DIY Beauty Recipes: Crafting Elixirs of Youth

The alchemical process of infusing ashwagandha into homemade beauty concoctions transforms the mundane act of skin and hair care into a ritual full of intention. A face mask, made with ashwagandha powder, honey, and rose water, becomes a potion that soothes, hydrates, and rejuvenates the skin, its application a moment of peace in the rush of daily life. Similarly, a cream, blending ashwagandha-infused oil with shea butter and essential oils, swathes the skin in a protective embrace, warding off dryness and imparting a radiant glow. Each recipe, part of nature's essence, offers the ability for people to control and improve their beauty regimen, connecting themselves to nature.

Hair-Care Applications: Reviving the Crowning Glory

Ashwagandha's foray into the hair care market unveils its capacity to nurture and fortify. The scalp, which is often neglected in the shadow of aesthetic focus on strands, benefits from ashwagandha's anti-inflammatory gifts, an intervention that soothes irritation and creates a fertile ground for hair growth. When incorporated into oils or shampoos, ashwagandha invigorates the roots, encouraging growth and bestowing the hair with volume and vitality. This botanical intervention, by addressing the root causes of hair health issues, offers a sustainable path to luscious locks, free from the traditional limitations of chemical dependency.

Safety and Patch Tests: Navigating With Care

While ashwagandha's topical application presents a panacea for various beauty concerns, the path to its integration into personal care routines demands caution. Everyone has different sensitivities, so conducting patch tests prior to widespread application underscores respect for these differences and acknowledgment of each person's distinct physiological landscape. A small amount of ashwagandha-infused product applied to a discreet skin area tests and gauges the body's receptivity and ensures the journey toward enhanced beauty avoids any unforeseen reactions. This cautious approach, coupled with vigilance toward any signs of adverse reaction, is all part of responsible engagement with natural beauty aids, ensuring that no harm is done.

Beauty can be superficial; ashwagandha goes beyond the superficial, with its combination of ancient and contemporary qualities, reflecting not just the external and its perceived perfection, but instead inner health and harmony. Ashwagandha invites a redefinition of beauty norms, advocating for practices that nurture the body's natural strength and radiance. Through the meticulous crafting of DIY beauty recipes, the integration of ashwagandha into hair care, and the observance of safety protocols, individuals can reap myriad benefits from the herb and its natural elements, cultivating an aesthetic expression that resonates with vitality and wellness, further confirmation of ashwagandha's enduring wisdom.

Special Precautions for Women: What You Need to Know

Application of ashwagandha requires a thorough, yet still nuanced, understanding. While lauded for its adaptogenic properties, this ancient herb can cause any number of complex interactions with a woman's hormones, necessitating caution to ensure its efficacy.

Hormonal Considerations

With the ebb and flow of hormonal effects defining much of women's health, ashwagandha steps in with a promise of balance. Yet, this promise is not without its caveats. For those in the throes of hormonal imbalances such as Polycystic Ovary Syndrome (PCOS) or thyroid disorders, ashwagandha's influence on endocrine function requires a measured approach. The herb's potential to modulate thyroid hormone production and possibly influence estrogen and progesterone pathways calls for a discerning application, tailored to individual hormonal contexts. It is through this meticulous customization that ashwagandha can be integrated into hormonal health management, offering support without disrupting the delicate balance.

Pregnancy and Breastfeeding

Pregnant and breastfeeding women should proceed with extra caution when it comes to herbal supplementation. There is currently a lack of conclusive research on ashwagandha and this phase of a woman's life. While traditional use advocates for its benefits, contemporary wisdom errs on the side of caution, suggesting abstinence due to a lack of any conclusive evidence on its safety. The counsel of healthcare professionals becomes indispensable, there to ensure that the choice to include or exclude ashwagandha from pre- and postnatal is as informed as possible.

Menstrual Cycle

The menstrual cycle stands as a barometer of overall health for many women. Ashwagandha, in its role as a modulator of stress and possible influencer of hormonal pathways, introduces variables into the menstrual equation that deserve attention. Observations suggest that while it may offer benefits in managing premenstrual syndrome (PMS) symptoms through stress reduction, its broader impact on the menstrual cycle remains a field yet to be fully explored. Mindful usage, attuned to the body's responses, allows for an integration of ashwagandha that respects the individual variability of menstrual health, ensuring that its introduction supports rather than disrupts.

Fertility

The quest for fertility, often marked by its share of challenges, finds a potential ally in ashwagandha. Preliminary research illuminates the herb's capacity to improve various markers of reproductive health, including hormone regulation and stress reduction, factors intimately tied to fertility. Yet, within this potential lies every woman's individual variability, where ashwagandha's effects are as unique as those making their way through this phase of their lives. A balanced perspective, grounded in both the optimism of emerging research and a cautious acknowledgment of the need for further study, guides the incorporation of ashwagandha into fertility protocols. This approach, coupled with the expertise of healthcare practitioners specializing in fertility, paves a path where ashwagandha is neither a miracle herb nor a panacea, but a potential piece in the complex puzzle of reproductive health.

In the field of women's wellness, where the interplay of hormones, life stages, and individual health narratives dictates a varied yet individualized approach to care, ashwagandha reminds us that it is rife with ancient wisdom navigating a modern landscape. Its application, marked by thoughtful consideration and a commitment to safety, mirrors the broader principles of holistic health—principles that encourage personalization, informed choice, and the integration of natural remedies within the spectrum of care. Through careful application and mindful observation, women can explore the potential benefits of ashwagandha, ensuring that its role in their wellness journey is both beneficial and harmonious.

Personalizing Your Ashwagandha Dosage

It goes without saying that everyone is different, each person having different physiological needs and health aspirations. Thus, discovering the optimal ashwagandha dosage becomes a pursuit of harmony. This quest, nuanced and deeply personal, relies heavily on body wisdom, scientific insight, and adaptogenic versatility, aiming to align the potent properties of ashwagandha with the singular narrative of one's health journey.

Finding Your Optimal Dose

Incorporating ashwagandha into your routine starts with the need to understand its potency and its potential impact on your well-being. Recommended dosages vary significantly depending on the source, from as little as 300mg to as much as 600mg of high-concentration extracts daily. This variability underscores the importance of starting with a conservative dosage, a necessary step as you and your body become attuned to ashwagandha's effects. It is in the attentive observation of your bodily and mental responses—be it an enhanced sense of calm, improved sleep quality, or a noticeable spike in energy— that learning what your optimal dose is and at which dosage your body responds best will occur. When you observe that your health goals are coming into clearer focus with help from ashwagandha's many benefits, you know you're on the right track.

Adjusting Over Time

As the seasons of life shift, bringing changes in stress levels, health conditions, and overall wellness goals, the ashwagandha dosage that once seemed a perfect fit may require recalibration. This fluidity is not indicative of a misstep but a reflection of the dynamic nature of health and well-being. An increase in life's demands, and therefore stress, for instance, may necessitate a slight uptick in dosage, leveraging ashwagandha's stress-mitigating prowess to maintain equilibrium.

Conversely, an enhancement in well-being, marked by stabilized stress responses and increased vitality, might signal a moment to taper the dosage, allowing the body to sustain its balance with a lesser quantity. This adaptive approach, responsive to the ongoing dialogue between ashwagandha and the body's needs, ensures the dosage remains in sync with the constant changes inherent to life.

Forms and Their Impacts

The confluence of ashwagandha's benefits with personal wellness practices extends into its various forms—powder, capsule, and tincture—each carrying nuances in absorption and effect. The powdered root, appreciated for its versatility, lends itself to culinary integration, offering a method of consumption that seamlessly piggybacks on daily routines, albeit with a slower absorption rate. Capsules, by contrast, present an easy convenience, their pre-measured doses providing clarity and simplicity, yet potentially distancing one from the tactile connection to the herb. Tinctures, potent and direct, offer rapid absorption, a sip of the herb's potency delivered with immediacy. This exploration of forms invites a consideration of lifestyle, preferences, and health objectives, guiding individuals toward a choice that resonates with their unique wellness path, ensuring ashwagandha's integration is as fluid as it is intentional.

Consulting With Professionals

Where ashwagandha's ancient wisdom meets the complexities of modern health profiles, the guidance of healthcare professionals becomes invaluable. This collaboration, particularly pivotal for those with chronic health wading through the pharmacological maze of medications, ensures ashwagandha's integration into one's wellness regimen amplifies rather than disrupts existing health strategies. A healthcare provider, armed with an understanding of ashwagandha's pharmacodynamics and an insight into the individual's health history, can tailor the dosage and form to optimize benefits while mitigating potential interactions. This partnership not only enriches the ashwagandha experience but also anchors it in a framework of safety and efficacy, a confluence of care that honors both the ancient origins of ashwagandha and the unique health journeys of those it seeks to nurture.

Adjusting ashwagandha's optimal dosage requires attentiveness, adaptability, and informed collaboration. This process, which reflects a broader pursuit of health and well-being, is not linear but cyclical, a continuous dialogue between individual needs, the evolving picture of health, and ashwagandha's potent adaptogenic properties. It is here, in the meticulous calibration of dosage and form, guided by professional insight and personal intuition, that ashwagandha's true potential is realized and integrated into daily life as a source of balance, vitality, and well-being.

Understanding the Market: Choosing Supplements Wisely

The quest for optimal holistic health can be a complicated affair— ashwagandha has emerged as part of a pathway to improved health and vitality, but the modern marketplace is an almost overabundance of choices. There are so many types of the herb in so many forms manufactured by so many companies that finding what is right for you requires a very discerning eye as well as an informed mind. How can you find the right product for you? Be informed and choose wisely.

Evaluating Brands and Products

The evaluation of various brands of ashwagandha requires scrutiny. Looks aren't everything, and it's easy to go straight for the most attractive packaging. But with ashwagandha, the ethos and practices underpinning the brand, as well as certifications, such as those from reputable organic and non-GMO verifying bodies, are worthier of your trust; they signal a commitment to standards that honor the purity of the herb and the sanctity of the environment from which it springs. Look beyond the labels and into the narratives of sourcing and manufacturing. Brands that cultivate transparent relationships with their cultivators and embrace methods that ensure the preservation of ashwagandha's potent compounds are clearly among those dedicated to excellence and efficacy.

Understanding Labels

The art of selecting the right ashwagandha supplement includes reading the label carefully; it will reveal the composition and concentration of the offering. Mastery of label literacy unveils the nuances between whole root powder and standardized extracts—a distinction critical in gauging the potency and therapeutic potential of the supplement. Seek out the concentration of withanolides, ashwagandha's primary active compounds, as a marker of potency. However, do not let this overshadow the holistic balance of the herb's phytochemical spectrum, for the synergy of compounds often transcends the impact of any single constituent. Furthermore, the discernment of excipients and fillers, those silent additions, underscores a commitment to purity—a prerequisite for those who place the sanctity of their bodies above all.

Avoiding Common Pitfalls

The journey through the supplement aisle is fraught with mirages and marketing ploys designed to enchant and ensnare. Beware the allure of buzzwords that promise miraculous cures and instantaneous transformations; true wellness comes from patience and consistency, not hyperbolic claims. The wisdom to distinguish between genuine, research-backed endorsements and flamboyant marketing tactics shields one from the seduction of baseless promises. Embrace skepticism while you wade through the options, allowing it to guide inquiries and investigations into the veracity of claims, ensuring that the choice of ashwagandha is evidence-based, not one caught up in the ephemeral allure of trends.

Ethical and Sustainable Sourcing

Be sure to deliberately seek out brands that clearly articulate a commitment to sustainable practices, brands that nurture the Earth as generously as it bestows the healing virtues of ashwagandha. This can be an act of defiance, righteously choosing social responsibility and environmental action over flashy siblings created for commerce and commerce alone. This act can also be a declaration of allegiance to the preservation of ecosystems and the land used to create this special herb. In trying to muddle through the market's vast expanse, armed with the discernment to evaluate, the wisdom to understand, the caution to avoid pitfalls, and the ethics to choose sustainability, the selection of an ashwagandha supplement goes beyond consumption. It becomes a declaration of values, to the belief in the power of nature to heal and the responsibility to do so in a manner that honors the Earth and its legacy. This journey, marked by the intent to infuse daily wellness with the purity and potency of authentic ashwagandha, is a pilgrimage to the heart of holistic health, a voyage informed by knowledge and guided by the principles of integrity and sustainability.

The Role of Ashwagandha in Detoxification and Cleansing

In our amazing bodies, where each cell plays its part in keeping us healthy, ashwagandha emerges as a silent leader, ushering in renewal and purification. This ancient herb offers its potent properties to aid in the body's natural detoxification processes, a gentle but powerful ally in the quest for purity and balance. With its roots deeply embedded in the soil of holistic wellness, ashwagandha extends an invitation to recalibrate and rejuvenate, supporting the liver's diligent efforts to cleanse the body of accumulated toxins.

A tireless guardian of health, the liver finds in ashwagandha a partner in its constant work, which is to filter and neutralize the myriad of toxins encountered in daily life. Ashwagandha's adaptogenic qualities are hard at work, mitigating the effects of stress on the body, a condition known to impede the liver's function. By easing the burden of stress, ashwagandha facilitates a more efficient detoxification process, allowing the liver to perform its duties with renewed vigor. Ashwagandha's support offers itself as a shield; also encourages the enhancement of the liver's inherent capabilities, a nurturing hand guiding the organ toward optimal performance.

Incorporating ashwagandha into detox routines requires an approach in line with the body's wisdom, advocating for methods that resonate with the principles of gentle cleansing. Integrating a daily dose of ashwagandha into a detox regimen, whether through teas, smoothies, or direct supplementation, introduces a layer of adaptogenic support that complements the body's efforts to purge toxins. This inclusion is a gentle, harmonious addition, aligning with the body's natural rhythms and enhancing the efficacy of detox practices without overwhelming the system.

Complementing ashwagandha's detoxifying prowess, a legion of practices and herbs stands ready to amplify the body's cleansing efforts. Hydration, a critical part of detoxification, works in tandem with ashwagandha, helping to eliminate the toxins through increased renal activity. Dietary choices, rich in antioxidants and fibers, act as allies, bolstering the body's mechanisms for dealing with free radicals and enhancing digestive function. Furthermore, the incorporation of other detoxification-supportive herbs, such as milk thistle for liver health and dandelion root for its diuretic properties, creates a synergistic blend that maximizes the body's detoxification potential. This holistic approach, merging together ashwagandha's benefits with complementary practices and herbs, embodies a comprehensive strategy for detoxification, one that respects the body's complexity and innate capacity for self-renewal.

The body's signals will guide you through detoxification, suggesting adjustments and tweaks to the regimen based on individual responses and needs. Attuning to these signals, whether they manifest as renewed vitality or temporary discomfort, informs the process of detoxification, ensuring it remains aligned with the body's pace and tolerance. This attentive stance not only optimizes the detoxification experience but also creates a deeper connection with your body, a dialogue that enhances understanding and respect for its needs and limits.

In this exploration of ashwagandha's role in detoxification and cleansing, the herb's adaptogenic capacity to support the body's purification processes is highlighted. From bolstering liver health to integrating seamlessly into holistic detox routines, ashwagandha easily aids balance and renewal. Complemented by many supportive practices and herbs, ashwagandha's inclusion in detoxification efforts illustrates a commitment to gentle, mindful cleansing, a path that honors the body's wisdom and innate healing capabilities.

As we close this chapter on ashwagandha's contributions to detoxification and cleansing, we're reminded of the broader implications of these practices for overall well-being. The journey through detoxification, supported by ashwagandha's adaptogenic strength, mirrors the larger quest for balance and health in a world where toxins, both physical and emotional, permeate our existence. This exploration, rooted in the ancient wisdom of Ayurvedic medicine yet deeply relevant to contemporary wellness challenges, invites a recommitment to holistic health practices that nurture and sustain. As we move forward, the insights garnered from ashwagandha's role in detoxification and cleansing serve as foundations for a deeper engagement with the natural world's healing gifts, a step on the path toward greater wellness explorations.

Review Request

Dear Reader,

Could you spare a moment to leave a review for this book?

Your review—which takes no more than a minute—could

- ignite a passion for a healthier and longer life for so many.

- inspire others to take this weight loss journey.

- transform someone's future just like you are transforming yours.

Imagine a life where your reflection in the mirror brings joy rather than despair, where every step you take feels lighter, and where you're in control of your relationship with food. That's the promise of *Ashwagandha: Secrets Revealed*. Now, you can share that hope and dream with others.

I'm calling out to you, my valued readers, to share your experiences and insights with the world. Your review has the power to inspire and guide others on their path to lasting weight loss. Together, we can reshape the narrative around health and vitality.

Ready to make that difference? Just scan the QR code below:

[https://www.amazon.com/review/review-your-purchases/?asin=BOOKASIN]

If the magic of sharing resonates with you, then you truly understand the spirit of *Ashwagandha: Secrets Revealed*. You are transforming yourself, and with a review, you can help transform others. This is my passion, and I know it can be yours.

Warm regards,

Chapter 4:

Ashwagandha and the Mindful Path to Wellness

In the quiet spaces between thoughts, where silence speaks volumes, a deeper understanding of wellness awaits. This space, often obscured by the din of daily living, holds the key to a form of well-being that goes beyond physical health, reaching into the essence of peace and mental clarity. Ashwagandha emerges as a guide to accessing this tranquil place, not through forceful intervention, but by harmonizing with the body's innate rhythms. Through the lens of mindfulness, where every moment is an opportunity for awareness, ashwagandha's role expands from a mere supplement to a catalyst for a deeper, richer connection with the self and the present.

Ashwagandha and Mindfulness: Enhancing Meditation Practices

Deepening Meditation Experiences

The act of meditation, a deliberate pause in the relentless flow of thoughts and activities, finds a powerful ally in ashwagandha. The herb's adaptogenic properties, known for tempering the body's stress responses, create an internal environment where the mind can more easily find stillness. Imagine the process of steeping tea; hot water slowly extracts the essence of the leaves, revealing the depth of flavor and aroma. Similarly, ashwagandha works over time to reduce mental noise and stress, enabling a deeper immersion into the meditative experience. The practice becomes not just a temporary retreat but a doorway to a more sustained state of calm and mental clarity.

Ritual Incorporation

Incorporating ashwagandha into premeditation rituals can significantly enhance the quality of the practice. A cup of ashwagandha tea, consumed in the quiet moments before sitting down to meditate, serves as both a physical and symbolic preparation, signaling the mind and body to enter a receptive state. This ritual, like laying out a welcome mat for tranquility, enriches the meditation experience, allowing for a more meaningful engagement with the present and a deeper exploration of the inner landscape.

Synergy With Mindfulness Practices

Ashwagandha's synergy with mindfulness practices extends beyond meditation; it will work its way into your daily life. Mindfulness, the act of being fully present and engaged with the here and now, benefits from the grounding effect of ashwagandha. The herb's influence on reducing stress hormones like cortisol not only ushers in a more mindful state but also enhances the body's resilience to day-to-day stressors. This partnership between ashwagandha and mindfulness practices creates a continuous cultivation of awareness, where each moment becomes an opportunity to connect deeply with the present.

Scientific Perspective

From a scientific standpoint, ashwagandha's support for neurological functions lays a foundation for effective meditation and mindfulness practices. Research indicates that ashwagandha promotes neuroplasticity, the brain's ability to form new connections and pathways. This adaptability is crucial for meditation, which relies on the brain's capacity to rewire itself, moving away from patterns of stress and reactivity toward states of calm and focused attention. The herb thus acts not only as a facilitator of immediate relaxation but also as a long-term ally in the journey toward a more mindful and centered way of being.

In this exploration of ashwagandha's integration with mindfulness and meditation, a path unfolds for those seeking not just relief from the symptoms of stress but a deeper, more enduring state of peace and mental clarity. This journey offers a holistic approach to wellness. It invites reconnection with the present, where each moment holds the potential for awareness, tranquility, and a deep understanding of the self. Through the mindful use of ashwagandha, individuals can navigate the complexities of modern life with kindness and compassion, embracing each day not as a series of challenges to be endured but as an opportunity for growth and deepening well-being.

Combating Modern Stressors With Ancient Wisdom

In modern times, stress has become a constant companion. This unwelcome guest, mostly created from societal expectations, technological inundations, and the relentless pace of life, insidiously undermines health and serenity. The modern way of life, with its unique stressors, from the ceaseless connectivity demanded by digital devices to the environmental and existential threats looming large, exerts a toll on the psyche and soma alike. It is within this context that ashwagandha's ancient wisdom can help lead you toward a better way of being, equilibrium, and tenacity.

The dialogue between the traditional uses of ashwagandha and its relevance in addressing contemporary stressors reveals an impressive continuity of human experience. Historically revered for its capacity to fortify the body against the many damaging effects of stress and strain, ashwagandha is as effective a stress reliever as it has been throughout history, despite the change in stressors. The herb, a harmonizer of the body's stress-response systems, remains a therapeutic salve for today's frayed nerves and continuous distractions

Incorporating ashwagandha into your daily routines is a practical strategy for stress management, a subtle yet potent recalibration of the body's response to external pressures. The morning, which so often can seem daunting, knowing the day ahead could be demanding or difficult, presents a perfect moment for ashwagandha's integration. A simple incorporation of ashwagandha powder into your morning smoothie or tea can set a tone of calm and fortitude for the day ahead. Evening, too, holds potential for ritualistic use; ashwagandha, taken in capsule or tincture form, can ease the transition into restorative sleep, unwinding the tension accrued through the day.

This strategic deployment of ashwagandha, however, goes beyond symptom management, aiming instead at reconstitution of the individual's relationship with stress. By modulating the body's cortisol levels and enhancing adrenal function, ashwagandha shifts the internal landscape from one of reactivity to one of resilience. Stress, under this new model, becomes not an overwhelming force to be battled but a challenge to be approached with logic and agility This change creates a state of balance in which you can manage life's many ordeals calmly.

Countless personal stories of people finding serenity and strength through ashwagandha confirm its efficacy and potency and how it helps through difficult phases of life. Consider the case of a high-powered executive, stuck in the relentless cycle of deadlines and demands, for whom ashwagandha could offer them a more centered presence, enabling a clarity of thought and calmness of spirit amidst corporate chaos. Or the story of a parent juggling the many pressures of work and family, finding in ashwagandha a source of sustenance, its use coinciding with a newfound ability to live through parenting's highs and lows with a steadier heart. These accounts, each unique yet unified in their theme of transformation, attest to ashwagandha's consistent relevance in providing solace and strength to those grappling with the stressors endemic to modern life.

The myriad strategies for integrating ashwagandha into the fight against modern stress are rich and varied, inviting a personalized approach to its application. For some, it may involve the ritualistic consumption of ashwagandha-infused beverages, a physical act of self-care that signals a commitment to well-being. For others, it may be the strategic use of ashwagandha supplements, a silent yet effective reminder of the body's capacity to fight back. And yet, for others still, it may manifest in the incorporation of ashwagandha into the kitchen, where the act of cooking becomes an alchemical process of turning stress into sustenance.

In this exploration of ashwagandha's role in mitigating modern stressors, a compelling narrative emerges, marked by a prudent yet meaningful application of traditional knowledge to modern challenges, illuminates a path toward wellness that is both attainable and sustainable. In taking advantage of ashwagandha's many virtues, individuals can feel secure and make the most of living in a modern, stressful world. They can feel a renewed sense of strength and peace. In this light, ashwagandha once again becomes a symbol of balance— looking at nature and balancing it with the modern world to create something so unique and effective.

Incorporating Ashwagandha Into a Plant-Based Diet

A plant-based diet, in which each ingredient is a testament to the Earth's bounty, ashwagandha finds a harmonious place. This ancient herb enriches the nutritional structure of a diet centered on plants, offering a bridge between the old world and modern dietary preferences. Recognizing the symbiotic relationship between ashwagandha and plant-based nourishment requires an appreciation for the varietal nutrients and natural compounds that sustain the body and spirit.

Nutritional synergies emerge when the adaptogenic qualities of ashwagandha amplify the inherent benefits of a diet rich in fruits, vegetables, legumes, and grains. The herb's capacity to modulate stress responses and support adrenal health complements the antioxidant and fiber-rich profile of a plant-based diet, creating a comprehensive approach to wellness that is greater than the sum of its parts. The interplay between ashwagandha and plant-derived nutrients builds an environment within the body that is resilient in the face of stress, vibrant in its energy levels, and grounded in a sense of well-being that permeates every facet of life.

With some creative culinary exploration, you can seamlessly blend ashwagandha into your diet of plant-based eating. Envision the morning ritual of blending a smoothie that combines the herb's earthy tones with the lush sweetness of ripe berries, the creamy texture of bananas, and the rich, nutty notes of almond milk. Here, ashwagandha transforms from a mere supplement into a culinary hero, enhancing the flavor profile while imbuing the beverage with its adaptogenic essence. Soups and stews can benefit greatly from adding ashwagandha while it simmers gently on the stove. A sprinkle of the herb's powder melds with the robust flavors of tomatoes, lentils, and spices, weaving its benefits into the heartiness of the dish without overshadowing the beautiful bounty of tastes that define plant-based cuisine.

The holistic health approach advocated by a diet rich in plants and the potency of ashwagandha resonates with the principles of balance and harmony. This nutritional philosophy does not merely aim to nourish the body in a physical sense but seeks to nurture a solid connection with the natural world, recognizing the interdependence of human health and the health of the planet. Ashwagandha underscores the importance of viewing dietary choices not as isolated acts of consumption but as integral components of a lifestyle that honors the body's natural rhythms and the Earth's ecological balance.

Environmental and ethical considerations infuse this integration of ashwagandha into a plant-based diet with a deeper significance, going beyond nutritional benefits to touch upon the stewardship of the planet. The conscious choice to embrace plant-based eating aligns with a commitment to sustainability, minimizing the ecological footprint associated with dietary habits. When ashwagandha's sourcing is approached with a similar mindfulness—prioritizing ethically harvested, organically grown, and sustainably sourced herbs—the act of consuming this adaptogen becomes a testament to a broader belief in environmental responsibility and ethical consumption. This alignment between dietary practices and ecological consciousness builds a sense of connectedness, a recognition that each meal, each herb, is a large part of life that thrives on respect, care, and reciprocity.

In plant-based diets, where ashwagandha intertwines with an abundance of natural foods, the journey toward wellness is more than simply eating. It becomes an exploration of how ancient wisdom, contained in a humble herb, can enhance modern dietary philosophies, enriching the body's health and the soul's tranquility. The incorporation of ashwagandha into this dietary framework is not merely about adding a supplement to a meal; it is about incorporating ancestral knowledge into contemporary life, creating a dietary pattern that is as nourishing to the spirit as it is to the body. Through this integration, the ancient and the modern converge at the dining table, inviting a deeper engagement with the foods we eat and the world we inhabit, a celebration of life's interconnectedness where each meal becomes an act of mindfulness, a gesture of respect for the body and the Earth.

Biohacking With Ashwagandha: A Guide for the Wellness Warrior

In the tricky maze of modern wellness, where technology meets ancient remedies, the practice of biohacking emerges as a call for those seeking optimization of the human body and mind. This pursuit, defined by a relentless quest to push the boundaries of human potential, blends the precision of science with the wisdom of age-old herbal traditions. Ashwagandha occupies a revered place as a friend of the biohacker, its roots deep in the fertile ground of ayurvedic medicine, yet its efficacy is celebrated in the cutting-edge field of contemporary biohacking.

Biohacking, in its essence, represents a big shift in our approach to health and performance. It is not merely about correcting deficiencies or combating ailments but about reimagining the limits of our biological potential. The goals are as varied as the methods, from enhancing cognitive function and emotional resilience to advancing physical endurance and longevity. Each biohacker composes a unique blend of interventions, lifestyle adjustments, and supplements designed to elevate their existence.

With this knowledge, ashwagandha emerges as a natural tool of remarkable versatility. Known for its adaptogenic properties, it addresses a core challenge in the biohacker's journey: the management of stress and optimization of energy. Modern society, full of psychological pressures and physical demands, often triggers a cascade of stress responses that can hinder cognitive function and impede physical performance. Ashwagandha, with its ability to modulate the body's stress hormones, introduces a countermeasure, a way to recalibrate our internal environment toward homeostasis. The result is a mind sharpened for mental endeavors and a body primed for physical feats, a duality at the heart of the biohacking ethos.

Strategies for integrating ashwagandha into a biohacking regimen abound, each tailored to individual rhythms and goals. The timing of supplementation, a critical consideration, hinges on the desired outcomes. Morning intake, for instance, can invigorate the start of the day, setting a foundation of resilience against stress to get you through the day. Evening doses, conversely, might help you unwind, preparing the body for restorative sleep, an often-overlooked pillar of peak performance. Dosage, too, demands attention, a balance struck between efficacy and sensitivity, often starting low and adjusting based on personal response.

Beyond its standalone use, ashwagandha's true potential in the biohacker's arsenal is realized in its combination with other biohacks. Synergies with dietary adjustments, fasting protocols, and nootropic stacks underscore its adaptability. Imagine, for a moment, the amplification of benefits when ashwagandha's stress-reducing power complements the cognitive uplift of a ketogenic diet or the enhanced focus derived from intermittent fasting. Such combinations exemplify the biohacker's art of synergy, a confluence of interventions that magnify health and performance outcomes.

The testimonies of individuals who have incorporated ashwagandha into their biohacking methods offer compelling stories of transformation. One such story unfolds with a software developer plagued by the twin specters of burnout and brain fog. The incorporation of ashwagandha, alongside a regimen of sleep optimization and mindfulness practices, marked a turning point. The fog lifted, replaced by a clarity of thought and a renewed vigor for innovation, a personal renaissance that underscores the impact of well-chosen biohacks.

Another account details the journey of an endurance athlete, for whom physical limits seemed an insurmountable barrier. The introduction of ashwagandha, in concert with targeted training protocols and nutritional adjustments, heralded breakthroughs in performance. Races that were once daunting became milestones of achievement, each finish line a nod to the power of strategic biohacking.

These stories, each unique in its contours, share a common thread: the pivotal role of ashwagandha in redefining the boundaries of mental and physical potential. They illuminate not only the herb's adaptogenic capabilities but also its place within the broader narrative of biohacking, where ancient wisdom and modern science converge in the pursuit of optimal wellness.

When it comes to biohacking, where every adjustment and supplement is a note in the symphony of self-optimization, ashwagandha plays a melody that resonates with the holistic nature of this pursuit. It is not merely a supplement but a bridge spanning the chasm between our ancestral heritage and our futuristic aspirations. Its integration into the biohacker's regimen exemplifies the fusion of past and present, a harmonious blend of nature's bounty and human ingenuity. As biohackers continue to discover the complexities of enhancing health and performance, ashwagandha stands as a steadfast ally, its roots anchored in tradition, its benefits radiating into the future.

The Science of Sleep: Ashwagandha's Role in Sleep Hygiene

When the quiet dark of nighttime arrives, myriad processes of restoration and healing occur. However, insomnia and disrupted sleep patterns can interrupt this important process. Stress and strain from today's modern life and all its demands don't offer much help. But within this context, ashwagandha can emerge as a mediator, offering you a more restful night of restorative slumber.

Role in Sleep Regulation

Understanding the details of sleep requires a comprehension of its architecture, a structure delicately constructed by the rhythms of the body's internal clock and the ebb and flow of neurochemical tides. Ashwagandha, through the lens of scientific inquiry, reveals its capacity to influence this architecture, enhancing sleep quality and regulating sleep cycles. Investigations into its pharmacological footprint uncover interactions with the GABAergic system, a neural pathway instrumental in inducing the calm necessary for sleep onset. This interaction, not unlike the gentle coaxing of the mind into a state of relaxation, underscores ashwagandha's efficacy in mitigating sleep latency and enhancing the depth of sleep, a boon for those wrestling with insomnia.

Practical Sleep Hygiene Tips

The incorporation of ashwagandha into the nightly routine shows off the herb's versatility and its adaptogenic alignment with the body's nocturnal rhythms. For optimal integration, a dosage an hour before bed, perhaps in the form of a soothing tea or a simple capsule, becomes a ritual, signaling to the body the impending descent into sleep. This practice, when coupled with other sleep hygiene rituals such as dimming lights to cue the body's circadian rhythm and creating a serene sleep environment, free from the harsh lights of electronic devices, transforms the bedroom into a sanctuary of rest. The result is a holistic approach to sleep, where ashwagandha acts not in isolation but as part of a concerted effort to honor and induce the body's natural propensity for rest.

Comparative Analysis

The modern market offers a plethora of sleep aids, each with its promises and pitfalls. Ashwagandha, when placed in comparison with these alternatives, both natural and pharmaceutical, distinguishes itself through a profile marked by safety and gentle efficacy. Unlike pharmaceutical options that may carry the risk of dependency and a myriad of side effects, ashwagandha offers a natural pathway to sleep, its adaptogenic qualities ensuring that its use supports the body's mechanisms for inducing rest without overriding them. Similarly, when juxtaposed with other natural aids, ashwagandha's broad-spectrum benefits, including its role in stress reduction and neuroprotection, afford it a unique position as a holistic sleep aid, addressing not just the symptoms but the underlying causes of sleep disturbances.

User Testimonials

Further proof of ashwagandha's impact on sleep is vividly painted in the testimonials of those who have found solace in it. Consider the account of an individual for whom the night was a battleground, sleep elusive and unyielding. The introduction of ashwagandha marked a turning point. Nights of restlessness gave way to a tranquility previously unknown, each morning a wonderful confirmation of uninterrupted sleep. Another narrative unfolds with a shift worker, her biological clock in constant flux, for whom ashwagandha became a stabilizing force, realigning her circadian rhythm, and restoring a semblance of normalcy to her sleep patterns. These stories, each a mosaic of personal struggle and triumph, illuminate the tremendous impact ashwagandha can offer sleep, proposing not just anecdotal evidence but a compelling case for its role in enhancing the quality of rest.

In the field of sleep science, where research and personal experience work together, ashwagandha's properties and potential emerge as a key player. This exploration, spanning the gamut from scientific inquiry to practical application, and comparative analysis to personal testimony, delineates a holistic view of ashwagandha's contribution to the nightly quest for rest. It highlights not just the herb's capacity to facilitate sleep but its role in enhancing the overall quality of rest, ensuring that the body and mind emerge from sleep rejuvenated and ready to greet the new day.

Ashwagandha and Relationships: Enhancing Emotional Well-being

When it comes to human relationships, emotions can take over at any time, and we find ourselves looking for some kind of balance. Because ashwagandha can help both physically and emotionally, it can offer us a path to better emotional regulation and strength, both of which we need to deepen our bonds and interact without stress and tension with the people we're closest to.

Emotional Balance

The chemistry of maintaining emotional balance in relationships, a task both delicate and daunting, finds an unlikely catalyst in ashwagandha. The herb's proficiency at modulating the body's response to stress indirectly creates an environment where emotions can be navigated with greater dexterity. Imagine the mind as a vast ocean, its surface whipped into furious waves by the winds of stress and anxiety. Ashwagandha, in this metaphor, acts as a balm, calming the tempest and allowing for clearer reflection and more nuanced emotional expression. This tranquility, hard-won in the constant clatter of daily life, becomes the bedrock upon which relationships can flourish, free from the stress that drags us down.

Enhancing Connection

Beyond the supporter of emotional stability, ashwagandha ventures into intimacy, both emotional and physical, its influence subtle yet profound. The reduction of anxiety and the elevation of mood work to build closeness in a relaxed presence. The herb's capacity to alleviate the undercurrents of anxiety that often besiege the mind paves the way for moments of connection, unmarred by our many worries and distractions. These moments, though fleeting, create a relationship full of shared joy and understanding and ashwagandha's effects are felt for a long time.

Communication and Conflict Resolution

In life there will always be some kind of conflict, where words spark rather than soothe; our need for resolution calls not only for empathy but for clarity. Here, again, ashwagandha's role surpasses the physical, greatly influencing communication. Where couples are struggling to resolve their conflicts or communicate effectively with each other, ashwagandha can help build clarity and give people the tools to solve these disagreements peacefully.

Personal Stories

Ashwagandha's impact on relationships has helped to write many personal stories, each a testament to the herb's transformative potential. Consider the narrative of a couple, their bond frayed by the incessant pressures of work and family responsibilities. The introduction of ashwagandha into their routine marked a turning point, the herb's calming influence acting to alleviate and counter the stress that had once threatened to unravel their connection. Conversations that once veered into contention now flowed into channels of constructive dialogue, one reshaped by a newfound peace.

Another tale unfolds with an individual for whom social interactions were minefields, each engagement fraught with anxiety. Ashwagandha, integrated into their daily regimen, served as a shield, softening the edges of anxiety and allowing for genuine connections to form. Social gatherings, once avoided, became positive opportunities for engagement, each interaction a step toward overcoming the barriers erected by fear.

These stories, each unique in its contours, come together on a singular truth: Ashwagandha, with its immeasurable effects on emotional well-being, holds the potential to redefine the dynamics of human relationships. When studying and looking at couples' improved emotional regulation, enhanced intimacy, effective communication, and the resolution of conflicts, ashwagandha emerges not just as a supplement but as a vehicle for deeper, more meaningful connections. In relationships, where the heart's resilience is both tested and celebrated, ashwagandha offers a road to harmony, helping us to define our interactions with those around us.

Sustainable Living With Ashwagandha: A Guide to Ethical Consumption

When looking at our planet and its interconnectedness at the heart of the world, ashwagandha becomes a symbol of this deeper connection. When approached with mindfulness and respect, its cultivation and consumption reflect this commitment to ethical choices and thoughts of what the future holds. This section will discuss how to integrate ashwagandha into our lives as more than a means for personal health. Doing so allows us to contribute to sustainable and ethical living.

Sustainability practices in the cultivation of ashwagandha reveal a plethora of methods that honor the Earth and its intricate ecosystems. The use of organic farming techniques, eschewing synthetic pesticides and fertilizers, ensures that the land remains fertile and the water clean, safeguarding the health of the planet and its inhabitants. Crop rotation, a practice as old as agriculture itself, maintains the balance of nutrients in the soil, ensuring that ashwagandha grows in harmony with the natural cycles rather than at their expense. Permaculture principles, applied to the cultivation of ashwagandha, create systems of agriculture that mimic the self-sustaining nature of wild landscapes, where every element supports the whole. Consumers, in their choice to support such practices, become custodians of a tradition that values the longevity of the Earth over the immediacy of profit, ensuring that the cultivation of ashwagandha contributes to the regeneration of our planet.

Ethical sourcing of ashwagandha goes beyond the mere transactional, evolving into an act of stewardship. It involves tracing the roots of the herb back to its origins, ensuring that it is grown and harvested under conditions that respect the dignity of labor and the sanctity of the Earth. Fair-trade certifications serve as markers of such commitments, indicating that farmers receive just compensation for their toil and that communities benefit from the commerce of ashwagandha. The choice of ethically sourced ashwagandha, then, becomes a statement, an affirmation of the belief in fair labor practices and equitable economic relationships. This conscious choice, made at the point of purchase, involves the consumer in a larger story of global justice and sustainability, where every product tells a tale of respect and reciprocity.

The broader impact of consumer choices on the environment and local communities producing ashwagandha invites a reflection on the action and reaction of every process. The demand for sustainably grown ashwagandha encourages farming practices that preserve biodiversity, ensuring that the fields where ashwagandha thrives are vibrant with life, a haven for pollinators and a refuge for soil micro-organisms. This demand also drives investment in rural communities, where the cultivation of ashwagandha can become a source of sustainable development, providing pathways out of poverty while respecting the cultural traditions that have nurtured the herb for generations. Thus, the act of choosing ashwagandha becomes an important part of a global ecosystem, where the health of the individual is inextricably linked to the health of the community and the vitality of the planet.

Living a sustainable lifestyle with ashwagandha at its heart invites a reimagining of our daily rituals and consumption patterns. It begins with a mindfulness about where our ashwagandha comes from, favoring sources that prioritize ecological health and social welfare. It extends to the way we consume ashwagandha, finding ways to integrate it into our diets that minimize waste and honor the herb's potency. From the repurposing of ashwagandha packaging into containers for seedlings to the composting of any residual plant matter, every action can reflect a commitment to a cycle of renewal and respect.

Furthermore, educating others about the benefits of sustainably sourced ashwagandha, sharing stories of its impact on health and well-being, becomes a form of advocacy, spreading the seeds of sustainability further into the community.

In this narrative of ashwagandha and sustainable living, a vision of consumption that is conscious and conscientious emerges, where the choices we make reflect a deep respect for the interconnected web of life. Ashwagandha, in this vision, is more than an herb; it is a symbol of our capacity to live in harmony with the Earth and to make choices that nourish not only our bodies but the world around us. Through the ethical consumption of ashwagandha, we participate in a story of renewal and hope, contributing to a future where sustainability and well-being are entwined, where every leaf and root reminds us of our covenant with the planet.

The Future of Ashwagandha: Trends and Innovations

The trajectory of ashwagandha's origins and efficacy is not only trending toward wider acceptance; it is full of potential, stretching out to reach the peak of human wellness and scientific inquiry. There is still so much to come—so many more discoveries through research, so many stories of its holistic success. The trajectory trends toward a future when ashwagandha will be widely accepted and integrated into our lives.

Current investigations into ashwagandha unfold across a wide variety of scientific disciplines, each peeling back layers to reveal new dimensions of its healing prowess. Neuroscientists continue to study its capacity to buffer the brain against the degenerative forces of age and disease, suggesting a future where ashwagandha is a foundation in the prevention of cognitive decline. Meanwhile, molecular biologists map the intricate pathways through which it modulates immune response, painting a picture of a future when ashwagandha's role in combating autoimmunity and bolstering our defenses against pathogens is well-defined and widely recognized. Each study illuminates the path toward a deeper, more nuanced understanding of ashwagandha's place in the pantheon of natural therapeutics.

Parallel to the myriad research is the constant uptick of innovation in product development. Ashwagandha, traditionally consumed as a powder or capsule, is being reimagined in forms that cater to the convenience and tastes of a modern audience. Effervescent tablets that dissolve in water, offering a refreshing beverage imbued with the herb's benefits, and highly concentrated liquid extracts that promise rapid absorption are at the forefront of a wave of products designed to integrate seamlessly into contemporary life. These innovations, each striving to balance fidelity to the herb's natural state with the demands for convenience and efficacy, sketch a future where ashwagandha's presence in our daily routines is as unobtrusive as it is useful.

The global market for ashwagandha reflects a burgeoning awareness of its value, a trend propelled by scientific validation and a collective yearning for wellness paradigms rooted in nature. Demand surges, drawing not only consumers but researchers and healthcare professionals into a growing conversation about how best to harness its properties. This dialogue, expanding across continents, cultures, and disciplines, shapes a marketplace where ashwagandha is both a commodity and a symbol of a global shift toward health practices that honor the wisdom of the past while embracing the possibilities of the future.

Predictions for ashwagandha's trajectory, informed by research, innovation, and market dynamics, envision an era where its role extends beyond the individual, becoming a major player in broader initiatives aimed at public health and wellness. Imagine community programs where ashwagandha becomes part of public-health strategies to enhance resilience against the pressures and pathogens that pervade our world. Or consider the potential for its integration into regenerative agriculture practices, where its cultivation supports not only the health of individuals but the health of the planet. This future, brimming with possibility, anticipates a time when ashwagandha's full potential is realized, part of a society that values wellness, sustainability, and the connections between human health and the health of the Earth.

As the curtain falls on this exploration of ashwagandha's future, it leaves us poised on the cusp of a new chapter in our relationship with this remarkable herb. The insights gleaned from emerging research, the innovations shaping its use, and the trends guiding its journey into the global market sketch a future rich with potential. This journey, marked by a fusion of tradition and innovation, promises not only to deepen our understanding of ashwagandha but to expand its role in our quest for wellness. As we turn our gaze toward the horizon, where the next chapter awaits, we carry forward the lessons of the past and the promise of the future, guided by the consistent wisdom of ashwagandha.

Chapter 5

Ashwagandha—The Cultural Codex

Ashwagandha's story is one of balance and rejuvenation. It's a vivid, fascinating, and old story, one that goes back to ancient India, allowing for a glimpse into the past as well as a means of studying the present and future of wellness. This herb has been around for hundreds, if not thousands, of years, and we still have much to learn from it.

Ashwagandha in Indian Culture: An Intimate Look

Historical Reverence

Tracing the roots of ashwagandha in Indian culture reveals a reverence that remains in place. In ancient Ayurvedic texts, it is celebrated not merely for its physical healing properties but as a conduit to spiritual awakening and balance. Consider the farmer in rural India, for whom planting ashwagandha is an act steeped in tradition, a rite that connects him not only to his ancestors but to the very essence of Ayurvedic philosophy. This herb, known as the "strength of the stallion," was believed to impart the vigor and vitality of a horse to those who consumed it, a testament to its highly valued properties.

Cultural Practices

The application of ashwagandha in traditional rituals and practices underscores its integral role in Indian culture and history. It finds its way into the sacred rituals of healing ceremonies, where its presence is believed to purify and protect, aligning the physical and spiritual health of participants. The use of ashwagandha in these ceremonies is not arbitrary but deeply symbolic, embodying the principles of harmony and balance that are at the heart of Ayurvedic medicine. It is in these moments of communal healing that ashwagandha transcends its physical form, becoming a bridge between the earthly and the divine.

Folklore and Myth

The folklore surrounding ashwagandha is as rich and diverse as India itself. Legends speak of sages who consumed ashwagandha to enhance their vitality and longevity, allowing them to meditate and perform rituals for years beyond the span of a normal human life. These stories, passed down through generations, do more than entertain; they weave ashwagandha into the cultural consciousness, embedding it in the collective memory of the people. The mythic qualities attributed to ashwagandha in these tales speak to its perceived potency and the respect with which it is regarded in Indian culture.

Modern-Day Relevance

Today, the relevance of ashwagandha in contemporary Indian society bridges ancient wisdom with modern wellness trends. In bustling city markets, vendors sell ashwagandha alongside a great many other herbs, a nod to the enduring popularity of traditional remedies despite the availability of modern medical advancements. Yet, it is not just in the markets that ashwagandha's presence is felt. Wellness centers across the country integrate ashwagandha into therapies and treatments, attesting to its adaptability and the growing recognition of its benefits in addressing contemporary health challenges. This resurgence is not a rejection of modern medicine but a harmonious blending of old and new, a recognition that health and wellness are multifaceted and that ancient wisdom still holds valuable insights for contemporary life.

In this exploration of ashwagandha within the rich cultural history of India, a picture emerges of an herb that is much more than a mere medicinal remedy. It is a symbol of balance, a bearer of tradition, and a bridge between the ancient and the modern. The reverence for ashwagandha in Indian culture provides a foundation upon which its global journey of wellness and healing is built. As we uncover the complexities of health in the contemporary world, the story of ashwagandha reminds us that wisdom often lies in the harmonious blending of tradition and innovation and that the roots of wellness run deep into the soil of culture and history.

Global Traditions: Ashwagandha's Role in Various Cultures

The global acceptance of ashwagandha is a testament to the herb's remarkable adaptability and the universal quest for wellness that goes beyond geographical boundaries. Its journey from the Indian subcontinent to distant lands is not merely a passage through space but a migration of knowledge, a validation of the herb's ability to ingratiate itself within a myriad of cultural contexts, each with its unique traditions of healing.

Cross-Cultural Adoption

The spread of ashwagandha beyond India marked the beginning of a fascinating chapter of herbal medicine. This dissemination was not a one-dimensional transfer of botanical specimens but a complex interchange of trade, exploration, and cultural exchange. In regions far removed from ashwagandha's origins, local healers and herbalists encountered the herb, recognizing in its vitality a reflection of their own traditions' reverence for nature's curatives. Thus, ashwagandha found a place within diverse medical systems, each adoption a reflection of the herb's versatile healing profile.

Comparative Traditional Medicine

When looking at traditional Chinese medicine, a system with its intricate theories of balance and energy, ashwagandha enters the pharmacopeia not as a foreign entity but as a familiar ally. Known as a qi tonic, it is valued for its capacity to strengthen the body's vital energy, seamlessly aligning with the principles of yin and yang. The parallels between this role and its use in Ayurveda as a vitalizer of life force underscore a shared recognition of the herb's essence across cultural divides.

Similarly, in the healing traditions of Africa, where the natural world is a potent source of medicinal knowledge, ashwagandha is embraced for its strength and ruggedness. African herbalists, attuned to the rhythms of the Earth and the healing powers it holds, integrate ashwagandha into practices aimed at fortifying the body against environmental and spiritual adversities. This integration speaks to a universal human endeavor to harness the natural world's restorative powers, a quest that ashwagandha has been part of for centuries.

Global Wellness Influence

The contemporary wellness field, a variety of practices drawn from across time and space, reflects ashwagandha's substantial impact on holistic health paradigms worldwide. In the West, where the hunger for natural health solutions has grown exponentially, ashwagandha emerges as a base of integrative wellness regimes. Its presence in supplements, nutritional plans, and therapeutic protocols is a nod to the herb's efficacy and the growing acknowledgment of traditional herbal wisdom as a vital component of modern health care. This global embrace of ashwagandha is not a trend but a convergence of historical ideas, a recognition that the pursuit of wellness is a shared human endeavor that benefits from a diversity of cultural insights.

Cultural Exchange

The journey of ashwagandha across the world's cultural landscapes is a story of exchange and enrichment. In this exchange, knowledge flows in multiple directions, allowing for a dialogue between traditional and contemporary, between East and West. Through workshops, academic collaborations, and online platforms, the wisdom surrounding ashwagandha is shared, scrutinized, and celebrated. This ongoing conversation not only broadens the herb's reach but deepens our collective understanding of its potential, building a global community united by a common interest in the healing powers of nature.

This dialogue is further enriched by the contributions of diaspora communities, who bring ashwagandha along in their journeys, seeding it in new soils, both literal and metaphorical. In doing so, they act as keepers of their cultural heritage while also participating in the global field of herbal medicine, illustrating the dynamic nature of cultural traditions as they adapt and evolve in response to new environments and discoveries.

Ashwagandha's global trajectory, from the ancient fields of India to the shelves of health food stores around the world, is evidence of the herb's enduring appeal and the universal human quest for health and balance. In its journey, ashwagandha has become a global citizen, a botanical ambassador that embodies the rich exchange of knowledge and traditions that enriches our collective pursuit of wellness. This narrative, created by countless tales of history, culture, and science, continues to evolve, propelled by ongoing research and the shared experiences of those who turn to ashwagandha for healing and harmony.

Personal Stories of Transformation: Ashwagandha Success Tales

In the fields of healing and personal evolution, the narratives that resonate most deeply are those of genuine experience and transformation. Ashwagandha has been a silent witness and facilitator of such metamorphoses, touching lives in myriad intimate ways. These tales, each a mosaic of struggle, discovery, and renewal, illuminate the herb's multifaceted role in boosting health, vitality, and equilibrium.

Health and Wellness Transformations

The journey of Elena, a graphic designer burdened by the relentless pace of her profession and the city's hum, mirrors the stories of many who find themselves adrift in the modern world's demands. For Elena, the discovery of ashwagandha was less about the pursuit of a cure and more about seeking harmony within a life that felt increasingly discordant. Initially skeptical, she integrated the herb into her morning routine, a simple act of self-care that gradually unfurled into a broader canvas of wellness. Over months, Elena noted a shift, subtle yet undeniable—a clarity of mind that allowed creativity to flourish, a sense of calm that turned stress into a navigable stream rather than an insurmountable barrier. Ashwagandha, for her, became a regular habit, a catalyst for a cascade of choices that nurtured her body and spirit.

Emotional and Mental Health

The narrative of Amir, a student navigating academia and the expectations of youth, speaks to ashwagandha's impact on emotional and mental well-being. Battling anxiety that was often so severe it was paralyzing, Amir found in ashwagandha an unexpected ally. The herb's grounding effect, subtle at first, grew into a foundation upon which he built layers of resilience. Study sessions no longer caused panic; examinations became challenges to be met with a steady hand and heart. Ashwagandha, in this context, fortified his mental health, allowing light to pierce through clouds of doubt and apprehension.

Physical Performance and Recovery

In the world of athletics, where every second shaved from a time and every ounce of effort exerted can delineate victory from defeat, ashwagandha holds many tales of strength and recovery. Consider the story of Lila, a marathon runner whose body began to betray her with injuries and fatigue that hinted of limits reached. Her introduction to ashwagandha came from a coach, a mentor attuned to the rhythms of natural healing. Integrating the herb into her regimen, Lila encountered not a sudden surge of power but a gradual accumulation of endurance, a resilience that saw her through training sessions and races. The herb's role in her recovery, aiding in the soothing of muscles and the calming of inflammation, marked a turning point, a stride toward achieving her athletic aspirations.

Chronic Condition Management

Chronic conditions are often marred by frustration and despair, but ashwagandha holds sway here, too. Sofia's tale, marked by rheumatoid arthritis, unveils the herb's potential in managing long-term ailments. Faced with a condition that gnawed at her joints and sapped her vitality, Sofia turned to ashwagandha as part of a broader approach to wellness that emphasized balance and holistic healing. The herb's anti-inflammatory properties offered not a cure but a means of coexistence with her condition, a path to reclaiming aspects of life once all but lost to pain and immobility. Ashwagandha, in this light, was less a medication and more a mediator, facilitating a dialogue between body and spirit that sought harmony rather than conquest.

These distinct narratives converge on a singular truth: that ashwagandha, through its myriad interactions with the human body and psyche, has the power to help people live better lives. The herb's journey across cultures and through time finds its most poignant expression in the personal stories of those it has touched. In these tales of health and wellness, emotional and mental resilience, enhanced physical performance, and the management of chronic conditions, ashwagandha reveals itself not merely as a supplement to be consumed but as a companion on the path to well-being.

The Community of Ashwagandha: Building Connections

In the vast, interconnected modern world, where digital platforms span the globe and bridge distant cultures, the community surrounding ashwagandha thrives. This herb, ancient in its roots yet modern in its application, has cultivated not just health and well-being but a vibrant collective of individuals united by their shared interest in its benefits. From online chat groups to silent labs and workshops, ashwagandha draws together those who seek not only healing but a better understanding of the natural world.

Online Communities and Forums

The digital age, with its unparalleled capacity for connection, has seen the emergence of numerous online spaces dedicated to the exploration of ashwagandha. These virtual forums buzz with activity, the herb's growing popularity bringing all walks of life together. Here, amidst the conversations, individuals from varied backgrounds share experiences, offering insights into the myriad positive effects of ashwagandha on their health and well-being. Questions posed by newcomers receive thoughtful responses, a reflection of the community's inclusive spirit and collective wisdom. Whether detailing the nuances of dosage and preparation or sharing personal stories of healing, these digital gatherings create a sense of belonging, a digital hearth around which enthusiasts and experts alike convene to exchange knowledge and support.

Local and Global Events

Beyond the screens, the community of ashwagandha enthusiasts extends into the physical world through events that celebrate and disseminate knowledge about this revered herb. Workshops led by herbalists, where participants learn to integrate ashwagandha into their daily routines, underscore the hands-on aspect of herbal medicine. Conferences on holistic health and wellness, meanwhile, often feature sessions dedicated to ashwagandha, highlighting the latest research and innovations in its application. These gatherings, whether local in scope or international, serve as communities of learning and connection, places where the theoretical meets the practical, and where individuals united by a common interest can interact, learn, and grow.

Collaborative Research Initiatives

The journey of ashwagandha from ancient remedy to modern superfood is paved with ongoing research, a collective endeavor that bridges continents and disciplines. Collaborations between universities, healthcare institutions, and independent researchers have given rise to studies that dive deep into the herb's pharmacological profile, exploring its potential in treating a wide range of conditions. These initiatives, often cross-cultural in nature, not only expand the scientific understanding of ashwagandha but also reinforce the connections between those who study it and those who use it. Through published studies, presentations at scientific symposiums, and participatory research projects, the community of ashwagandha researchers contributes to a growing body of knowledge that informs and enriches the global discourse on herbal medicine.

Support Networks

At the heart of the ashwagandha community lies the support network, a network of relationships built through shared experiences and mutual aid. For many, the ashwagandha experience begins with a search for healing, a path often fraught with uncertainty and challenges. Within the community, however, individuals find not just information but empathy, a collective reservoir of encouragement and advice that sustains them through their explorations. Support groups, both online and in person, offer spaces for individuals to share their struggles and triumphs, creating an environment in which healing is a communal journey. These networks, characterized by their nonjudgmental and nurturing ethos, exemplify the community's underlying philosophy: The pursuit of health is a collective undertaking, enriched by the diversity of its participants and sustained by their shared commitment to wellness.

Ashwagandha and Spirituality: Exploring the Deeper Connections

Ashwagandha has an immeasurable capacity to nurture the human spirit. More than an herb, it blurs the boundaries between self and the divine, a spiritual messenger that speaks a quiet, soulful language to anyone willing to listen.

The spiritual significance attributed to ashwagandha finds resonance across a spectrum of meditative and yogic disciplines, where the herb is viewed not just as a means to enhance physical vitality but as a tool for spiritual awakening. Its role in these practices is varied, deepening meditation, enhancing the focus required for yoga, and fostering a state of mindful presence that invites spiritual insights. The adaptogenic qualities of ashwagandha, which bring balance to the body's physiological processes, similarly extend to the spirit, harmonizing the internal energies that influence our states of consciousness. This harmony, essential for the pursuit of spiritual growth, allows practitioners a view of their inner worlds with a clarity and tranquility that enhances their spiritual practice.

In the sanctified spaces where rituals and ceremonies bridge the human with the divine, ashwagandha assumes a deeply sacred role. Its inclusion in rituals across various spiritual traditions is not a matter of coincidence but a recognition of its revered status and its perceived ability to purify, protect, and connect. Burning ashwagandha as incense during sacred ceremonies, for instance, is believed to cleanse the aura, creating a conducive environment for spiritual encounters and divine communion. Similarly, the ingestion of ashwagandha before meditative practices is thought to strengthen the mind-body connection, ushering in a state of receptivity to spiritual experiences.

The exploration of the mind-body connection, a cornerstone of holistic wellness, finds in ashwagandha a potent ally. The herb's adaptogenic prowess, renowned for its ability to mitigate stress and build physical equilibrium, similarly nurtures the mind, preparing it for the rigors of spiritual exploration. This preparation is critical, for the journey into the spiritual often demands a tenacity and openness that is best supported by mental and physical well-being. Ashwagandha, by enhancing this connection, acts as a facilitator of spiritual awareness, encouraging a mindfulness that is both grounding and expansive. It is in this state of heightened awareness that individuals find the capacity to explore the depths of their spirituality, encountering insights and understandings that are transformative.

Personal spiritual journeys, intimate odysseys of discovery and enlightenment, are markedly enriched by ashwagandha's presence. Accounts abound of individuals for whom it has been a companion on the path to spiritual awakening, its use coinciding with periods of great personal growth and insight. One such narrative involves a seeker who, in the midst of a spiritual lull, turned to ashwagandha as part of a broader quest for renewal. The herb's calming influence, coupled with its ability to enhance focus, became a key that unlocked deeper levels of meditation, revealing layers of consciousness previously unexplored. Another recounts the experiences of a yogi who found in ashwagandha the strength to sustain the physical demands of rigorous yogic practices, leading to an elevation of their spiritual practice. These stories, personal yet universal, highlight the diverse ways in which ashwagandha supports the spiritual journey.

In this exploration of ashwagandha's spiritual dimensions, the herb emerges as a bridge between the tangible and the intangible, the physical and the metaphysical. Ashwagandha, in its essence, invites a deeper engagement with the spiritual aspects of existence, offering tools for exploration and growth that are rooted in the ancient wisdom of herbal medicine. This engagement opens avenues for spiritual exploration that are rich with potential for enlightenment and transformation. In the world of spirituality, ashwagandha stands as a guide, a nurturer of the spirit, and a catalyst for the deepening of practices that connect us to the world within and the world beyond.

Q&A With Experts: Demystifying Ashwagandha

In an environment where nature and science collide, ashwagandha emerges as a botanical enigma, satisfying both the curious and the scholarly. To understand its benefits, applications, as well as its potential, a dialogue with experts in herbal medicine, Ayurveda, and nutrition becomes imperative. This conversation, a confluence of perspectives and expertise, seeks not only to illuminate the depths of ashwagandha's properties but also to dispel the mists of doubt and misconception that often cloud its understanding.

Within this assembly of knowledge, questions posed by those seeking to integrate ashwagandha into their lives find answers grounded in both tradition and empirical evidence.

Expert Insights

The discourse begins with an exploration of ashwagandha's *adaptogenic nature*, a term that, while now part of the wellness lexicon, demands elucidation. Experts elucidate this concept, describing adaptogens as botanical agents that strengthen the body's resistance to stressors, enhancing its ability to maintain equilibrium despite any physical and emotional challenges. Ashwagandha epitomizes this adaptogenic capacity, offering a shield against the strains of stress while cultivating an environment of internal balance.

Addressing Misconceptions

Misconceptions about ashwagandha, ranging from its effects to its application, pervade public consciousness, requiring clarification. One such misconception lies in the belief that ashwagandha serves as a quick fix, a magical elixir that offers immediate relief. Experts counter this notion, emphasizing the herb's role as part of a holistic approach to health, one that requires patience and consistency. The benefits of ashwagandha, they assert, manifest gradually, its effects building over time, nurturing resilience and vitality rather than providing instantaneous solutions.

Practical Advice

The conversation then meanders into practical application, addressing the questions that linger in the minds of those looking to add ashwagandha into their lives. On the matter of dosages and forms, experts advise a tailored approach, one that considers individual needs and responses. The versatility of ashwagandha, available in powders, capsules, and tinctures, allows for flexibility in its incorporation into daily routines. For those seeking to optimize its benefits, the timing of intake emerges as a focal point of discussion. Mornings may welcome ashwagandha for strength and vitality when facing the day ahead, while evenings embrace it as a step toward peaceful sleep.

Future Research Directions

The dialogue culminates in a forward-looking discussion on the frontiers of ashwagandha research, where the promise of future discoveries looms large. Experts speak of ongoing studies aimed at unraveling the herb's molecular mechanisms, its interaction with the body's myriad systems, and its potential role in addressing chronic conditions. The exploration of ashwagandha's impact on cognitive health and its capacity to support mental well-being in an age marked by increasing psychological stressors stands at the forefront of scientific inquiry. This research, burgeoning in its scope, heralds a future where ashwagandha's contributions to health and wellness are both broadened and deepened, highlighting its potential.

Through this dialogue, the complexities of ashwagandha are unraveled, its benefits illuminated, and its future potential cast in the light of anticipation, marking a path for exploration and understanding in the continuous journey toward holistic well-being.

The Art of Growing Your Own Ashwagandha

Growing ashwagandha at home continues a long-standing tradition of ancient hands eager to nurture the herb. Growing it at home, far from being a mere cultivation of a plant, emerges as taking part in the cycle of growth, offering insights into the rhythms of nature and the sustenance it provides. In the cultivation of ashwagandha, one finds not just the growth of an herb but the flourishing of a relationship between the gardener and the garden, a dialogue that spans seasons and speaks of patience, care, and reciprocity.

Home Gardening Tips

Opting for seeds of high vitality ensures a strong start, a foundational step toward a bountiful harvest. Planting, timed to coincide with the gentle warmth of spring, allows ashwagandha's roots to root deep into the earth, seeking nourishment and stability. The soil, prepared with care to achieve a blend rich in organic matter, becomes the seeds' precious home, waiting for potential growth. Watering, a common ritual of sustenance, is moderated to meet the herb's modest needs, avoiding the extremes of drought and saturation. This balance, a key to thriving growth, mirrors the equilibrium ashwagandha bestows upon those who seek it for healing.

Understanding Growth Conditions

Ashwagandha's resilience finds its roots in the optimal conditions under which it thrives. This herb, accustomed to the dry terrains of its native lands, seeks the warmth of the sun, basking in its rays to gather the energy required for growth. The climate, ideally warm yet not scorching, invites ashwagandha to stretch toward the sky, its leaves capturing the light, its roots anchored in the cool earth below. Soil, the foundation of growth, is chosen for its light texture and nutrient richness, a medium through which roots can navigate freely. Water is administered with a mindful approach that reflects the natural rainfall patterns ashwagandha is accustomed to, ensuring that the plant's needs are met.

Harvesting and Processing

As seasons change and ashwagandha has maximized its growth, the time for harvesting begins, a period of reaping that rewards the patience and care invested. The roots are unearthed with reverence. Leaves, too, bear the imprint of healing, harvested in their prime to capture the full spectrum of their benefits. The process of drying, a bridge between harvest and use, is undertaken with an eye toward preserving the integrity of the plant's compounds, a slow surrender of moisture that concentrates its healing essence. Grinding, the final step in the change from plant to powder, is done with a mindfulness that honors the journey from seed to sustenance, yielding a form ready to be integrated into daily wellness practices.

Sustainable Practices

In the cultivation of ashwagandha, the gardener becomes a steward of the Earth, a role that carries with it the responsibility of nurturing not just a plant but the environment that sustains it. Composting, the act of returning to the Earth what was borrowed, enriches the soil, fostering a cycle of growth that is regenerative and sustaining. Water conservation, a practice that reflects the herb's modest needs, becomes a principle adhered to with diligence, utilizing methods that minimize waste and maximize efficiency. Crop rotation ensures that the soil remains vibrant and alive, capable of supporting growth for seasons to come. In these practices, the cultivation of ashwagandha transcends the boundaries of gardening, becoming an engagement with principles of sustainability that echo the herb's ethos of balance and harmony.

The art of growing ashwagandha confluences tradition, wisdom, and environmental stewardship, a journey that extends beyond the confines of the garden into personal and planetary well-being. This endeavor offers not just the tangible rewards of harvest but also the intangible benefits of engagement with the Earth and its offerings.

Crafting Ashwagandha Beauty Products

Where personal care is concerned, ashwagandha reveals its versatility not just as a guardian of internal well-being but as a potent ally in the field of aesthetics. This ancient herb lends itself to the creation of beauty products that do more than adorn or embellish. They serve as conduits for the herb's restorative essence, enhancing the natural radiance of skin and hair. Herein lies an invitation to embrace it as a key ingredient in the art of creating beauty products that nurture and rejuvenate.

DIY Beauty Recipes

The crafting of ashwagandha-infused beauty products at home unfolds as an exploration of creativity and personal care, a journey into the heart of herbal cosmetics. The foundation of this endeavor is a collection of recipes, each a testament to the herb's adaptability and efficacy. A facial serum, combining ashwagandha's extract with oils of jojoba and rosehip, promises not just hydration but a defense against the environmental stressors that besiege skin daily. For the scalp and hair, a treatment blending ashwagandha powder with coconut oil and lavender essence offers nourishment, strength, and a soothing fragrance, addressing the roots to tip in a holistic embrace. The creation of a face mask, combining the herb with clay, turmeric, and honey, becomes a ritual of purification and renewal, drawing out impurities while bathing the skin in ashwagandha's protective essence.

Natural Skincare Benefits

The integration of ashwagandha into beauty regimens is underpinned by a synthesis of scientific findings and herbal medicine, a confluence that illuminates the herb's benefits for skin and hair. Research delineates its antioxidant and anti-inflammatory properties, mechanisms through which it combats oxidative stress and inflammation, culprits of aging and degradation at the cellular level. Traditional applications, observed across cultures, speak to its use in promoting a complexion that is not only clear but radiant, and in nurturing hair that exudes vitality. This duality of action, protective and restorative, positions ashwagandha as a cornerstone of natural beauty care, offering a pathway to aesthetics grounded in health.

Personalization Tips

The craft of formulating ashwagandha beauty products is inherently personal, a dialogue between the individual and the ingredients that acknowledges the uniqueness of every skin and hair type. Tailoring these creations demands an attentiveness to one's needs and responses, an exercise in intuition and observation. For those with skin leaning toward dryness, the addition of moisturizing agents like shea butter to ashwagandha face creams can provide an extra layer of hydration. Conversely, for oilier complexions, the incorporation of astringent elements such as witch hazel refines the formulation, balancing oil production. In hair care, the customization extends to addressing specific concerns, be it enhancing volume with aloe vera or combating dandruff with neem oil, always with ashwagandha at the center.

Eco-Friendly Packaging

Crafting ashwagandha beauty products at home extends beyond the personal to the environmental, a recognition that true beauty care is as much about nurturing oneself as it is about honoring the planet. This philosophy finds expression in the choice of eco-friendly packaging and storage solutions, a commitment to sustainability that complements the natural purity of the products. Glass jars, with their timeless appeal and endless recyclability, emerge as ideal vessels for serums and creams, while biodegradable tubes offer a green alternative for balms and masks. The selection of these materials, each a small act of conservation, adds an eco-conscious element to the practice of herbal beauty care, aligning the personal ritual of adornment with the broader ritual of environmental stewardship.

Staying Informed: Continuing Your Ashwagandha Journey

The pursuit of knowledge regarding this ancient herb is not a path tread lightly but a voyage steeped in the commitment to understanding its depths, nuances, and evolving applications. This dedication to staying abreast of the latest scientific explorations and scholarly discourse on ashwagandha demands a strategy that is both meticulous and expansive, ensuring that one's engagement with the herb is informed, reflective, and grounded in a comprehensive appreciation of its potential.

At the heart of this endeavor lies the imperative to wade through the massive amounts of research around ashwagandha, a task that requires both discernment and curiosity. Academic journals and scholarly articles illuminate the cutting edge of ashwagandha science, from clinical trials elucidating its therapeutic effects to molecular studies unraveling its complex bioactive constituents. These resources, often dense with data and analysis, demand a patient and critical eye, allowing for the extraction of insights relevant to both the practitioner and the lay enthusiast. Engaging with this body of work creates not only a deeper understanding of ashwagandha's mechanisms and benefits but also an appreciation for the rigor and precision that characterizes contemporary herbal science.

Parallel to the scholarly exploration of ashwagandha is the quest for educational materials that bridge the gap between academic research and practical application. Books authored by experts in herbal medicine and Ayurveda offer a wealth of knowledge, weaving together traditional wisdom and modern scientific findings into a coherent narrative. Websites dedicated to herbal wellness, chock full of articles, guides, and product reviews, serve as accessible platforms for expanding one's knowledge base. These resources, curated with an eye for credibility and depth, provide a foundation upon which individuals can build their understanding and appreciation of ashwagandha, integrating its use into their wellness regimens with confidence and insight.

The cultivation of community engagement stands as a pillar of the ashwagandha journey, a dynamic interchange of experiences, knowledge, and support that enriches one's relationship with the herb. Online forums and social media groups offer myriad personal narratives, practical advice, and scholarly discussion, creating a space where enthusiasts and experts alike gather to share and learn. Local workshops and seminars, often hosted by herbalists and health practitioners, provide an opportunity for hands-on learning and direct interaction, building a sense of connection and community among participants. This engagement, vibrant and multifaceted, underscores the communal aspect of herbal medicine, a shared endeavor that transcends individual experience and contributes to a collective reservoir of knowledge and wisdom.

At its core, the journey with ashwagandha represents a broader commitment to lifelong learning, a recognition that the landscape of herbal medicine is ever-evolving and rich with discovery. This commitment demands an openness to new information, a willingness to question and explore, and a dedication to integrating newfound knowledge into one's practice and understanding. It is through this continuous process of learning and exploration that the full spectrum of ashwagandha's potential can be appreciated—not only as a therapeutic agent but as a catalyst for personal and collective growth in the realm of wellness.

As this chapter on ashwagandha draws to a close, its varied role in herbal medicine encourages inquiry, education, and community engagement. The journey with ashwagandha, marked by a dedication to staying informed, engaged, and open to research trends and tradition, reflects a broader narrative of wellness that is dynamic, interconnected, and rooted in the rich soil of knowledge and exploration. In this narrative, ashwagandha serves not merely as a subject of study but as a companion on the path to understanding health, wellness, and the healing power of nature. As we turn our gaze forward, the insights gleaned from this journey illuminate the way, guiding us toward new horizons of health and harmony in the chapters to come.

Conclusion

As we draw the curtains on this enlightening journey through the world of ashwagandha, you should pause and reflect on the ground we've covered together. From its deep roots in ancient tradition and culture to the forefront of modern holistic wellness, ashwagandha has revealed itself as a spotlight of health, strength, and harmony. The synthesis of its rich history, its health benefits spanning the physical, mental, and emotional, and its practical applications for daily use underscore its role as a cornerstone in the pursuit of well-being.

The universal appeal of ashwagandha, bridging the gap between ancient wisdom and contemporary science, cannot be overstated. Its adaptogenic qualities, offering a shield against stress and a pathway to vitality and longevity, present ashwagandha as a versatile tool accessible to all, regardless of age, lifestyle, or health status. This book has woven together transformational stories, underpinning the immense personal and community impact of this remarkable herb. These testimonials serve not just as narratives of change but as inspiration for you, the reader, illustrating the tangible benefits of integrating ashwagandha into your life.

However, as we embrace ashwagandha's gifts, let us do so with mindfulness toward quality, sourcing, and sustainability. Your choices matter—opting for ethically sourced, sustainably farmed, and high-quality ashwagandha ensures that we honor this herb's legacy while minimizing our environmental footprint. And while ashwagandha stands as a powerful ally in wellness, it shines brightest when part of a holistic approach to health, complementing a balanced diet, regular exercise, mindfulness practices, and adequate rest.

I encourage you to continue exploring, learning, and experimenting. Engage with communities of enthusiasts and practitioners, stay abreast of the latest research, and dare to integrate ashwagandha into your wellness routines. Let this book be your springboard into the vast ocean of natural wellness, with ashwagandha as your guide.

To you who stand at the threshold of this voyage, I say, start your ashwagandha journey today. Whether it's through integrating a supplement into your daily routine, experimenting with ashwagandha-infused recipes, or delving deeper into its history and benefits, take that first step. Remember, the path to wellness is as unique as you are, and ashwagandha offers a flexible, supportive companion on your quest for health and happiness.

In closing, I extend to you not just the knowledge contained within these pages but my heartfelt belief in the transformative power of ashwagandha and natural wellness. My passion for helping others achieve optimal well-being inspired me to write this book. It is my sincere hope that it serves as a valuable resource on your journey to health and happiness. Remember, you are not alone. A vibrant community, including myself, stands ready to support you as you explore the enriching path of ashwagandha and holistic wellness.

Embrace the journey, for it promises to be as rewarding as the destination itself.

References

An Overview on Ashwagandha: A Rasayana (Rejuvenator ...
https://www.ncbi.nlm.nih.gov/pmc/articles/PMC3252722/

An Overview on Ashwagandha: A Rasayana (Rejuvenator ...
https://www.ncbi.nlm.nih.gov/pmc/articles/PMC3252722/

A Prospective, Randomized Double-Blind, Placebo ...
https://www.ncbi.nlm.nih.gov/pmc/articles/PMC3573577/

A Prospective, Randomized Double-Blind, Placebo ...
https://www.ncbi.nlm.nih.gov/pmc/articles/PMC3573577/

A Prospective, Randomized Double-Blind, Placebo ...
https://www.ncbi.nlm.nih.gov/pmc/articles/PMC3573577/

A Prospective, Randomized Double-Blind, Placebo ...
https://www.ncbi.nlm.nih.gov/pmc/articles/PMC3573577/

Ashwagandha: Is it helpful for stress, anxiety, or sleep?
https://ods.od.nih.gov/factsheets/Ashwagandha-
HealthProfessional/

Ashwagandha (Withania somnifera)—Current Research on ...
https://www.ncbi.nlm.nih.gov/pmc/articles/PMC10147008/

Ashwagandha (Withania somnifera)—Current Research on ...
https://www.ncbi.nlm.nih.gov/pmc/articles/PMC10147008/

Ashwagandha for Sleep https://www.sleepfoundation.org/sleep-
aids/ashwagandha

Ashwagandha Powder For Skin - DIY Recipe for Skin Whitening
https://www.vedaoils.com/blogs/news/ashwagandha-powder-
for-skin

Can Ashwagandha Benefit the Endocrine System?—A Review
https://www.ncbi.nlm.nih.gov/pmc/articles/PMC10671406/

Combining Adaptogens: A Guide
https://dragonhemp.com/blogs/learn/guide-to-combining-adaptogens

Effects of Ashwagandha (Withania somnifera) on Physical ...
https://www.ncbi.nlm.nih.gov/pmc/articles/PMC8006238/

Efficacy of Ashwagandha (Withania somnifera [L.] Dunal) in ...
https://www.ncbi.nlm.nih.gov/pmc/articles/PMC4687242/

4 Ashwagandha Recipes for Your Adrenals
https://www.banyanbotanicals.com/info/blog-the-banyan-insight/details/4-ashwagandha-recipes-for-your-adrenals/

Good Agricultural Practices for Ashwagandha - DMAPR
http://www.dmapr.org.in/Publications/bulletine/Good%20Agricultural%20Practices%20for%20Ashwagandha.pdf

In the mood for ashwagandha: 2022 Ingredient trends ...
https://www.nutritionaloutlook.com/view/in-the-mood-for-ashwagandha-2022-ingredient-trends-for-food-drinks-dietary-supplements-and-natural-products

I Took Ashwagandha For One Year, Here's What Happened
https://medium.com/the-mood/the-most-powerful-herb-you-never-heard-of-1ffe0ff3c2fe

Organic cultivation of Ashwagandha with improved ...
https://www.ncbi.nlm.nih.gov/pmc/articles/PMC5901777/